Praise for Kelley and Thomas French's

JUNIPER

"An extraordinary memoir."   — O, *The Oprah Magazine*

"Raw, rough, and wrenchingly tender. Two parents, flawed in many ways, very different from each other, have written of a singular experience that is presented with such grace it is an almost universal story of love and determination and strength."
— Sharon Peters, *USA Today*

"Beautifully written...it will stay with you long after you finish."   —Carla Rohlfing Levy, *Good Housekeeping*

"A well-told, fast-paced, and emotionally affecting memoir."
—Terri Rupar, *Washington Post*

"These two excellent journalists bring their keen eyes to the most personal and wrenching of stories. A powerful book."
—Tracy Kidder

"*Juniper* is a tender, fierce, and breathtaking miracle."
—*People*

"This surprising, enlightening book transcends categories. Heartfelt as a memoir, richly researched as narrative journalism, and as propulsive and literary as a novel, *Juniper* offers the rewards of all great books. It alters and expands your understanding of being human."
—Sheri Fink, author of *Five Days at Memorial*

"Two skilled journalists collaborate on the most personal of stories: their extremely premature daughter's struggle to survive....A fierce and fact-filled love story with few holds barred." —*Kirkus Reviews*

"Kelley and Thomas French are two of America's best narrative journalists, and here is their most important story yet. *Juniper* is an astonishingly intimate and honest account of a mother, a father, and a complicated baby whose very existence calls into question every easy assumption about what a life means. This is a deeply moving and meaningful book."
                —David Finkel, Pulitzer Prize–winning journalist
                        and author of *Thank You for Your Service*

"This tender account is vividly rendered, with husband and wife writing alternating chapters, so the story is told from different perspectives, and in distinct voices, but with a shared energy and urgency." —*National Book Review*

JUNIPER

JUNIPER

The girl who was born too soon

Kelley and Thomas French

Back Bay Books
Little, Brown and Company
New York Boston London

Back Bay Books / Little, Brown and Company
Hachette Book Group
1290 Avenue of the Americas, New York, NY 10104
littlebrown.com

Originally published in hardcover by Little, Brown and Company,
September 2016
First Back Bay paperback edition, October 2017

Back Bay Books is an imprint of Little, Brown and Company,
a division of Hachette Book Group, Inc.
The Back Bay name and logo are trademarks of Hachette Book Group, Inc.

The publisher is not responsible for websites (or their content) that are not owned by the publisher.

The Hachette Speakers Bureau provides a wide range of authors for speaking events. To find out more, go to hachettespeakersbureau.com or call (866) 376-6591.

Photographs on pages ix, 5, and 57 are courtesy of the authors. All others are courtesy of Cherie Diez.

The lyrics on page 265 are from "Waitin' On a Sunny Day" by Bruce Springsteen.
The lyrics on page 285 are from "That's the Way That the World Goes 'Round" by John Prine.
Kelley's prayer for Juniper on page 214 is borrowed from Tina Fey's "Mother's Prayer for Its Daughter" in *Bossypants*, © copyright 2011 by Little Stranger, Inc.

ISBN 978-0-316-32442-7 (hc) / 978-0-316-32443-4 (pb)
LCCN 2016933403

10 9 8 7 6 5 4 3 2 1

LSC-C

Printed in the United States of America

For Junebug

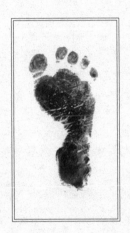

We are unfashioned creatures, but half made up,
if one wiser, better, dearer than ourselves—such a
friend ought to be—do not lend his aid to perfectionate
our weak and faulty natures.

—Mary Shelley, *Frankenstein*

Contents

Authors' Note

This is a work of nonfiction, based on our family's experiences at All Children's Hospital in St. Petersburg, Florida, and our reporting there in the years since. Nothing has been invented. Almost all of the scenes are based on notes we took during our daughter's stay in the neonatal intensive care unit. We checked our notes and recollections through interviews with many of the doctors, nurses, and nurse practitioners who cared for our daughter and through our review of her seven-thousand-page medical chart.

JUNIPER

The Tunnel

She arrived at the edge of what is possible and what is right, the shadowland between life and death, hubris and hope. Her eyes were fused shut. The plates of her skull were half formed, leaving her head more squishy than solid. Her skin was so translucent that just below the surface we could see the shuddering fist of her heart.

The doctors and nurses ringed her plastic box, summoning all of their arts and deploying all of their machines, working at the limit of human capability to keep her with us. We soon forgot what day it was, what we had been doing before we arrived in this place—our jobs, our plans, the vanities that had defined us. We'd been dropped inside a tunnel and were down so deep there was no way back.

She was perpetually dying, then not dying, then dying again. Slowly, we discovered that the only escape was to create a world for her beyond the box. So we filled her endless night with possibilities and sang her songs about the sun and read her books in which children could fly. We shared the story of how we had fought to make her ours. We told her the parts that humbled us, the moments that broke us. The frailties and failings that conspired against her creation.

If we made her long to know what happened next, maybe we could keep her with us until dawn.

PART ONE

Creation

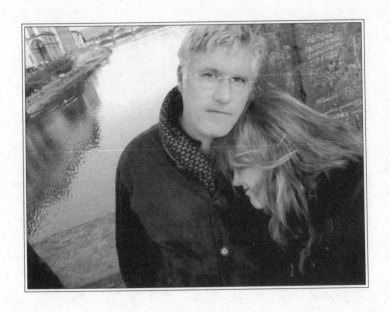

Kelley

Fallen creatures should not always be rescued. I have always known that, and yet. When I was fourteen, a friend offered me a baby bird, cupped in her palms. She'd found it among the pine needles in the Florida horse pasture where we spent our days.

His body was a blue heap of twigs wrapped in rice paper, threaded with veins and sugared with fuzz. His bobblehead teetered on a stalk of a neck, and his sealed eyes bulged blindly. His mouth was a gaping maw of need.

He was exotic and thrilling. In my suburban backyard, I had defended the naked rat babies in the compost pile from the threat of my father's shovel, begged for the lives of the raccoon family in the attic. I'd raised stray kittens in the garage, puppies in the family room, and bunnies on the back porch. So that day, when my mom picked me up, I climbed into her old red Ford Falcon holding a shoe box and not expecting her to object. My parents had plenty of flaws, but their gift to me was the freedom to explore.

I was finishing my freshman year of high school. I was awkward and often alone. I knew this bird was, in the scheme of things, not special. But his heart fluttered in my hands. I carried him into the living room and set him up in an old, cracked aquarium I found in the garage. I put in a branch or two from the magnolia in the yard, a sad attempt to make his habitat more natural.

It's probable that someone asked what was the point. Even if I saved him, he couldn't live in our house, like a parakeet, and he couldn't go free. Those were distant concerns. I soaked chicken feed in warm water and offered it every couple of hours in a syringe. It slid down his throat with a satisfying glug. I felt the divide between the civilized and the wild. Wasn't I barely civilized myself, always bumping into invisible boundaries, finding the shape of the world? I was powerless in the halls at school, powerless over my too-big teeth, my disobedient hair, and my dad, who decapitated the baby rats in the compost pile, blasted the raccoons out of the attic with a .22 rifle, sold my puppies, gave away my bunnies, and took my kittens to the pound.

This bird's small life, whatever it would become, was in my hands. I would protect him as long as I could. The next day, his lashless eyes peeled open. The first thing he saw was me, staring at him through the glass.

The bird grew fast. He sprouted feathers in tufts and stalks. He morphed into a bright, squawking blue jay. He lived in my bedroom, far enough from the main living area of the house that I got away with it, for a while. He perched on my ceiling fan, and I put the daily *St. Petersburg Times* underneath to catch the poop. Every morning he landed on my chin and tap-tap-tapped on my nose with his beak. Wake up. Wake up. Wake up. He drank Coke from the rim of my can. He pecked at birdseed and scraps of my dinner, which I often ate in my room, alone. He liked to perch on my shoulder or on top of my head, clutching with his dinosaur feet. Sometimes he caught rides on the back of our pug dog, Wrinkles, who was too dense mentally and physically to object. I'd take him outside and he'd visit the scrub pines, but he always came back to my shoulder. I hoped strangers would see us and believe I had magical powers. I felt like I did.

Eventually my mom said I had to let him go. He'd often find me on my walk to school and ride on my head part of the way there or back. After a few weeks, I came home and found him dead on the back porch. I guess I'd broken him in ways I couldn't foresee. He'd had nowhere else to go, no other safe place to land.

I grew up. I had dogs and horses. I smelled of hay and dirt. I imagined that someday I'd have a farm, with room for all the wild or broken baby things. I knew also, even though I never babysat or played with dolls, that I'd have a daughter.

She would be fierce and wild and dirty and drag a kitten under one arm. She would climb trees and sing. I would not forget what it was like to be a kid and to love something warm and alive. I would not forget how it felt to be afraid—afraid to make friends, to dance in public, to be seen at the beach, to talk in class, to bring home a boy. I'd protect her wildness. She'd bring home a stray cat or a rabbit or a baby bird. I'd show her how to care for it, to protect its wildness. I'd teach her when and how to let go.

It was a certainty, not a wish. When I was little, I'd asked my mom how you got a baby. She said, "Well, first, you have to want one." She didn't explain further, so I guess it stuck in my mind that the wanting was the only essential ingredient. The wanting was what mattered.

When our daughter was born—after everything went wrong, and the certainty turned to longing and the longing drowned out everything—she looked just like that baby bird. She was knobby, papery, translucent, and blind. Not all fallen things should be rescued, I understood. But no one was going to say no if we wanted to try. Who was more helpless, her or us? Her toothless mouth gaped in need. We stared at her through a wall of glass.

To understand the improbability of her, the odds against that first breath, we must go back to that summer I raised the blue jay. Because that was also the summer I met Tom, who had a small but crucial cameo in my teenage life. I've wrestled in the years since with the absurdity of it all. Because even if the story had ended there, it would have been strange enough.

Tom was one of the speakers at a high school journalism camp I attended. He was a hotshot reporter in his thirties, married with two small boys. I had been reading the *St. Petersburg Times* since the fifth grade. I loved the mischief in his columns railing against school administrators who would censor high school journalists. I loved the compassion and ambition in his book-length series about a murdered woman in Gulfport. His stories were daring and absorbing, like novels. I swooned over his byline: Thomas French.

He wore a purple shirt and zebra-striped shoelaces that day, which was off-putting. His glasses swallowed his face. His hair, dark and floppy across his forehead, was already turning gray. He was sweet, but he was a nerd, which I found somehow reassuring. I had no self-confidence, and though people told me all the time that I was a good writer, I knew they were just being kind. Tom had insecurities, too. He kept swigging Diet Coke and glancing out the window and running his hands through his hair. His nerves somehow made the work he was doing seem more achievable.

He told us to see past authority figures with their titles and their passive-voice pronouncements and unearth the unofficial story, the real story, bubbling under the surface. He told us to take the reader into the "secret garden"—the back of the nail salon, the corner of the teachers' lounge, the places where collusions were formed and power was transferred. Real stories did not arrive via press release. They did not announce themselves, but they were all around us, for the plucking. He told us our interests were not trivial. The things we cared about mattered. We mattered.

I wrote about him that day. In the paragraph that journalists call the nut, which is supposed to distill the thing to its essence, I wrote: *He never does anything halfway.*

I didn't fall in love, break up his marriage, and steal his children. That would have been absurd, and a felony. But I changed. I opened up. I started noticing the beauty in small details, the sublime in the everyday. Those lessons stayed with me, became part of me.

I graduated from high school, started college, and interned in the summers at the *St. Petersburg Times*. I fell in love, a few times.

Rick was first. I loved him like a drug. But after three years I left him because I knew he'd never have kids. It shouldn't have mattered yet; I was just twenty-two. But my wild little girl was already real to me. Next came Bill—my brilliant and soulful journalism professor. When I moved to south Florida to take a teaching job, I let him slip away. Then came a chiseled and easy-going personal trainer, whom I left for grad school, and a series of interchangeable D.C. intellectuals. I broke up with one because he was too skinny and another because he sweated too much.

When I found Tom again, I was twenty-eight. I hated dating, bars, and men in their twenties. I was finishing grad school in Maryland and trying to land a job at the *St. Pete Times*. Tom was in his early forties. He had won a Pulitzer Prize, gotten divorced, and ditched the glasses. His face was leaner, his hair almost silver. His boys were in elementary school. He had a longtime girlfriend who was older than him. "A sweet woman," he called her.

We had dinner when I went to Florida for a job interview. It wasn't a date, but he was so easy to talk to it started to feel like one. He talked on and on about how he still wanted a daughter. I picked at my trout as my ovaries did somersaults. He still had that openness I remembered. He baked cookies. He volunteered in his boys' classrooms and hand-made their Halloween costumes. He wasn't afraid to talk about hard things. He was the exact opposite of most of the men I'd ever known. Dinner lasted four and a half hours.

I e-mailed my friend Lucia: *I would marry him, end of story. He gave me a hug at the end, and I can smell him in my hair.*

We had a crazy chemistry that caught me by surprise, because he was wrong in so many ways. He was too old, too short, too divorced. He disliked animals, dirt, vegetables, exercise, unfamiliar foods, home repair, and the outdoors. He was emotional and overly sensitive. He talked too much. And the girlfriend.

That summer he came up to Baltimore to teach at a nearby college. I drove over and watched him lecture about writing using Monet. He explained how the artist observed the transformation of the Rouen Cathedral in the shifting light of the passing sun and how, on the page, respecting the natural sequence gives a story shape and power. When I was around Tom, I felt like I was bathing in a different light.

The next day, I met him again, and before we could leave his hotel for dinner, he launched into an angsty discussion of our by-now-undeniable mutual attraction, invoking his girlfriend by name. "I am a nice guy," he said. "But I am human, and I am not married." *Shut up,* my brain was screaming, the attraction dissipating. "So I have to make a decision and" — Christ, was he still talking? — "and I want you to respect —"

I kissed him to make him stop talking. To make him forget the girlfriend, or any previous or concurrent women, or any version of himself that had ever existed that was afraid to begin again. I kissed him to say, *If you never do this again, you'll miss it for the rest of your long, static life.*

"Why me?" he asked hours later, hair and shirt all a mess. Whatever I'd done had not calmed his insecurity. He seemed love drunk, sure, but lost.

I did my best to answer. He was interested in the world, its history, its richness, its forces and counterforces. All its crazy beauty became magnified and reflected in him, and when I was around him, it rained on me.

I saw him the next day and the next. Driving home one afternoon I was overwhelmed by the urge to pee. I pulled over at the National Cathedral, where surely they had clean bathrooms. I walked around inside that place, a temple to the things man can build and the things beyond his understanding, the afternoon sun streaming through stained glass. Man's filter and God's light. A service was starting, so I hung around. I wasn't religious, but I was in love, and that felt like religion. I lit a candle. When I left, the light had changed again. It was foggy and dark, and I thought of Tom, the world spinning around him, exerting its forces, and I hoped that inside him, something would move.

Over the next few months, I moved to Florida and started my job, and tried to allow the tension to build. Tom would call, late. I came to expect it.

"You're like this vast, unexplored continent," he said one night on the phone. "And I could wander around it forever."

He paid attention. He listened. He remembered the things I said and tried his best to make sense of them. With him, I grew more aware of myself. Everything that mattered to me—love, writing, parenting—began with a heart in a conversation. He was good at that. He was better at that than anyone I had ever known.

"Writing is a concentrated form of paying attention," he told me. "And so is singing, and kissing and praying."

He said he loved me. He said he was going to break up with the girlfriend, but then he didn't. He didn't want to hurt her. He needed to "understand."

"I think too much," he told me.

"I can't split myself in two," he said.

"I have told myself I need some time."

Weeks turned to months turned to years. At work, I wrote about a rooster attack, a garbage-truck race, and a man who spent twenty-six years on death row. I got promoted twice and landed my dream job on the feature staff. My new boss, Mike Wilson, was one of Tom's closest friends and fast becoming mine, too. I had a cubicle with a window, and I could see Tom from my desk.

I bought a four-bedroom house that I shared with my neurotic, emotional Weimaraner, Huckleberry. The house was too big, and the emptiness made me feel more alone. I spent all of my spare time nesting. I scraped paint, built a fence, planted bird-of-paradise. I replaced doorknobs, hinges, siding, molding, light fixtures, fans. I hung a swing from the branch of a broad live oak. I knew where the nursery and tree house would go.

I fostered puppies for the local animal rescue. Whatever it was in me that had once wanted to save that blue jay had swelled. By now I'd fostered hundreds of puppies for four different shelters in three cities. My mom, who lived nearby, would bottle-feed them and talk to them and cradle them belly up in her arms like furry grandbabies.

Tom faded in and out as I drew him in and pushed him away. He bought a cramped cinderblock house that I hated—a clear sign, I told myself, of our incompatibility. While he dithered, I dated other fine, available, confident, attractive, dog-loving, baby-wanting men. I always stopped returning their calls. I was stuck.

Ex-Boyfriend Number One, Rick, put it to me plain. "You know who you ought to marry?" he asked one day on the phone. "Tom French."

Ugh, I told him. That guy's a disaster.

Tom was the one I wanted, though. I couldn't will myself to want anything else.

I refused to believe that the frightened, scattered version of himself he presented to me was real. Inside that shell was a guy who didn't just love Springsteen, he had seen him in concert seventy times, always up front, screaming the lyrics. He couldn't just write a story, he had to write a nine-part series that took five years. In things that mattered, he chose to commit. *He never does anything halfway.* Even my fifteen-year-old self had known this.

I stubbornly believed, as so many women believe about so many men, that I could help him rediscover the best parts of himself, the person he might have been had divorce and middle age not beaten him blind.

I wanted my kids to talk to me like Tom's sons talked to him. I wanted to watch Nat and Sam grow up. I wanted my kids to share their love of Shakespeare and *South Park*. They were already two of the finest humans I'd ever met—generous and joyful and funny. Tom was damaged, but they were perfect. And he was part of the reason.

I watched Tom sing with them as they incorrectly loaded the dishwasher with unrinsed plates. He overlooked the patches in the mostly mowed lawn. He bought out the first three rows for their performance in *Urinetown*. Together, they debated the narrative arc of *Battlestar Galactica, Team America,* and the gospel of the Boss. The kitchen forever smelled of bacon, and the floor stuck to my feet. It all melded into an exuberant mess that I could imagine as my life.

One night after work, not thinking, I turned in to his neighborhood. The street was a circle, and I wandered around it for a while, wondering what in the hell I was doing there, until, suddenly, I was passing in front of his house. It was December, and the blinds were open in the front windows, and the light was warm inside. Nat and Sam were at the dinner table, and Tom and the girlfriend were sitting down to join them.

What did you expect, stalker? This is not your family. Find your own goddamn family.

I hated myself. I had wasted so much time. I spent another Christmas with my parents. My mom worked that morning. When I woke up, the house was empty.

Almost imperceptibly, Tom turned cold on the subject of more kids. He had a million reasons, none of which made sense. At first I brushed it off, because of course he wanted more kids, but he retreated behind some invisible shield.

He made me playlists full of promises, and I'd sing along in my car, searching for meaning, and then I'd find duplicates on his computer, made for other women. He spent long hours on the phone with God-knows-who. I kept asking him who she was. He always lied.

"Listen," Rick said. "You tell that motherfucker you are not going to beg."

My counselor said I should move on, buy sperm from a bank, have a baby on my own. It started to not seem crazy.

Tom slept too easily, always with his back to me. I could never sleep, lying next to so much confusion, so I'd just watch him breathe. With my finger, I'd slowly trace messages on his back, all the things I couldn't say, as it rose and fell and rose and fell.

I—L—O—V—E—Y—O—U

Asshole.

Tom

In the beginning, I saw Kelley only in secret, at midnight. My official girlfriend lived an hour north of Tampa, which made it simple to steal away. She was a kind and faithful woman who would have done anything for me. Late at night, I would call and tell her about my day and listen as she told me about hers, and then I would tell her I loved her and taste the ashes of those words in my mouth.

Speeding down the interstate toward Kelley's bed, I would put on the faraway face I wore whenever I knew I was committing a sin but was not ready to feel the shame. Kelley lived at the other end of the county, which meant there was always too much time to reflect. Usually I waited until I was on the Bayside Bridge, skirting north over Tampa Bay, before I called to tell her I was on my way.

"Where are you now?" she would ask.

"Maybe fifteen minutes away."

"What would you do if I said no?"

When she said this, I'd stare out at the pavement rushing toward me, the pelicans swooping in and out of the shadows, the black water stretching on either side. She wasn't about to stop me, and both of us knew it. I heard the anger in Kelley's voice, and below that an awful sadness. She was better than this and couldn't understand why I was not. But I also could hear that my brashness satisfied something in her. She wanted me to claim her. She was biding her time, hoping that I would redeem myself with a ring, a house, a baby. That was the problem. I had worn a ring once, for many bitter years. The only good things to come out of that marriage had been Nat and Sam. They were growing up fast and would soon be headed for college. I could not see the point of starting over.

Behind the wheel of my SUV, I turned up the stereo to shut out my brain. On these midnight drives, I gravitated toward dreamlike songs of isolation. The Stones and "Moonlight Mile," Springsteen quietly vanishing into a pitch-black night in "Stolen Car." What I listened to the most was Beth Orton's *Daybreaker*, the desolation in her voice, the sense of someone who had gone too far and would never be the same. How much damage was I causing, especially to myself? Despite my distrust in marriage, I yearned for the simplicity of the vows. I was hopeless at being single. I did better with clear-cut rules, a handbook written by God. Though I had long since drifted from my Catholic upbringing, the nuns lived on inside my head.

By now I would be off the bridge and turning onto Sunset Point Road, cutting west past the darkened fronts of taquerias and gun shops, past convenience-store parking lots where teenagers lingered in the neon clouds emanating from the Budweiser logos in the front windows. Halfway down there was a little strip mall, the Time Plaza, with a big clock out front that had stopped working. Every time I drove by, I held my breath and asked myself if it were possible for me to have died without knowing it.

Just beyond the turnoff for Kelley's street, there was a flashing yellow light. When I spied it in the distance, I clicked ahead to the last track on *Daybreaker,* "Thinking About Tomorrow," and sang along with Orton as she told her lover farewell, even though she was made for him and created for him. Good-bye, so long, so long. This was our song, Kelley's and mine. She just didn't know it yet.

She was always waiting when I arrived, a vision materializing in my headlights. She would stand in front of her big glass front door, her long brown hair falling soft over her shoulders. Neither of us said a word. I could never get over the way she folded into my arms.

I said as little as possible, and explained myself not at all. These late-night visits weren't just lust, I was sure. I had never been wired for superficial experiences and had no interest in flings. Though I had no right to say such things, I told Kelley over and over that I loved her and tasted the ashes of those words, too, even though they were true.

In the middle of the night, I would wake and feel her breathing against my shoulder. I wanted to stay forever. I wanted to leave right away. The dog, Huck, had the good sense not to trust me. When I stirred and headed for the bathroom, he would wake and stalk me with his yellow eyes. Sometimes he growled. Once, he padded over and blocked my path. I was wearing only a T-shirt, and before I knew it, he had lightly fastened his teeth through the bottom of the shirt and onto my crotch, daring me to move. A second or two later, he let go.

That morning, when I told Kelley, she laughed.

"Huck didn't bite you," she said. "If he'd wanted to bite you, he would have."

She was staring at me now, no longer smiling.

"Besides," she said, "you deserve it."

She always told the unvarnished truth. At the newspaper,

when I showed her early drafts of my stories, she wouldn't say, "I can see what you're going for here." She would toss the print-out on my desk and say, "Um, it went on too long. You're doing that wordy thing again."

There was nothing nice about Kelley, at least nothing she carried around like a badge. She didn't care about self-promotion. In my head I kept a list of her quiet acts of kindness. She volunteered at an elementary school and mentored a fifth-grade girl. She had donated bone marrow, simply because there was a shortage. I knew about her work with unwanted dogs, of course, and how she had stolen a starving Doberman from a crack house. She brought pregnant dogs into her guest room and helped them birth their puppies. One night, she'd delivered ten German shepherds, and then when she realized more puppies were stuck inside the mom, she had reached in and pulled out four more squirmers and given them mouth-to-nose resuscitation, breathing them back to life.

Kelley was always rescuing vulnerable creatures. Especially pit bulls. She felt a kinship with powerful animals. She often spoke of how much she wanted to touch a tiger. In those days I was reporting on the zoo in Tampa and following the keepers who watched over two Sumatrans. Kelley asked if I could arrange an encounter. Maybe she could pet one.

"A tiger," I said, studying her face for some hint that she was joking. "You'll be lucky not to lose an arm."

"I would be careful. I would only pet the tiger for a second."

She was a puzzle I could never solve. She did not seem to need anything, except what I would not give her. Though she made her living with words, she was not a big talker. Sometimes I would ask her a question, and fifteen minutes would pass before she answered, usually in a pronouncement of crystalline concision. Mysterious and self-contained, she refused to be understood before she was ready. The only time I avoided conversation was late at night, when Kelley asked me when the hiding would finally end.

"You know, you don't have to figure this out all by yourself," she said. "I wish you'd let me in there with you."

It was sobering, cataloging our differences. Kelley wanted to cuddle apex predators. I had been afraid of animals, especially dogs, ever since some bad experiences when I was a young paperboy. Kelley was handy around her house, constantly fixing doors and shelves with an arsenal of power tools. I could barely hammer a nail. Her grandfather had once slapped her grandmother for voting for a Democrat. My grandfather had once gone to confession for voting for a Republican. Our writing styles were just as dissimilar. My writing overflowed with detail. Kelley's stories were so spare that they left the reader to fill in the blanks. On the page, as in her life, she remained just out of reach.

Kelley was thirty, now ready to begin a life. I was forty-six and still recovering from the wreckage of my marriage. I could not understand Kelley's insistence that the two of us were meant to be together. So much of her faith in me was tied up in my skills as a dad.

"I've seen your work," she said. "I know what you can do."

There was no denying that I was wired for fatherhood. The oldest of five siblings, I'd been training for the job since I was a kid. Even as a boy, I had imagined myself grown up and holding a little girl in my arms.

When my first wife gave birth to our first child, I was so sure it would be a girl that I could not believe my eyes when the nurse held up the red and squirming baby. *What the hell is that between my daughter's legs?* I thought.

When Nat and Sam were babies, I balanced them on my shoulder and danced them to sleep. After the divorce, the boys and I grew even closer. They had a beautiful and unbreakable bond with their mother, but now my time with them was mine alone. I woke them up with songs from *The Wizard of Oz* and showed them how to cook in our little kitchen. Sometimes the hamburgers fell apart before reaching the buns. The omelets were usually too runny, or scorched. Didn't matter.

Nat and Sam were still in preschool when I taught them the words to "Thunder Road" and "Badlands." I coached them on how to yowl like Wilson Pickett and hoot like the Beatles. We worked especially hard on the little yelp McCartney breaks into as Lennon plows through the second verse of "Bad Boy." There was a whole world inside that one raucous cry, and I wanted my boys to claim it. I wanted them to be wild and strong and know that they were never alone.

Our days and nights were defined by stories. On rainy Saturday afternoons, I showed them *Star Wars* over and over. On the playground, when I pushed them on the swings, we pretended we were X-wing pilots attacking the Death Star. As the boys grew, they became obsessed with Harry Potter. The first books in the series were just coming out, and when each installment was released, they would beg me to buy two copies so they could devour them simultaneously. From age eleven onward, they repeatedly checked the mailbox, hoping for their invitation to Hogwarts.

Beyond my parenting skills, I could not fathom why Kelley wanted me. I wasn't as clever as her or as good a writer. I wasn't as charming or as smart or talented as other serious boyfriends she'd had. The best I could do was take her to a movie and then show her how to map out the story, scribbling the sequence on a napkin at the Greek restaurant down the street. "I know it's an A/B structure," she'd say impatiently. "Can we just eat?"

In the morning, when I shuffled into the bathroom, I barely recognized the man gazing back at me in the mirror. The lines of exhaustion, spidering around the eyes. The bewildered expression of someone perpetually playing catch-up.

Something inside me was broken. I worried that I only knew how to skate the surface of things, that I had never learned how to hold on to anything that counted, or to even recognize what counted. I suspected that I was not a person at all, but a facsimile of a person. A forgery.

"You know, you don't have to pretend with me," Kelley said. "I don't need you to be perfect. I just need you to be yourself."

What could I say? I wasn't even sure how to summon that person. I doubted that either of us would like him, whoever he was.

In December, two and a half years after I started seeing Kelley, I broke up with the official girlfriend. Kelley was suspicious, and who could blame her.

For the next six months, we went through the motions of becoming a couple. We raked the leaves in her front yard, walked Huck together, got barbecued ribs from a food truck parked in front of the convenience store down the street. I played her *Born to Run* and would catch her softly singing the lyrics in the car, her head turned away because she was self-conscious about her voice. On weekends when Nat and Sam were around, she laughed as they mocked me and plotted with them to convince me that they needed a trampoline, despite my fears of emergency-room visits.

The four of us were already strategizing about Halloween. Nat and Sam and I were planning a party, and Kelley helped us brainstorm. She had given me a little gargoyle statue, a winged dog in chains. According to the package, he was the Guardian of Hopes and Dreams. I had several life-size skeletons, and two mummies that I positioned every year in the front window, with a candle casting flickering shadows on their gray faces. Kelley one-upped me by ordering a skeleton of a dog from a veterinary-supply catalog.

She was a natural with the boys, not pressing for their affection, easing into the seams of their lives. But I grew increasingly certain that I was too old for the life she envisioned. I saw us standing at the altar and then her getting pregnant and promptly dumping me. She would be granted custody of the baby and would bankrupt me with child support and alimony, just as I was approaching retirement. I tortured myself with visions of leaning on a cane as I inched along the sidelines of youth soccer games, a stooped and wheezing specter. I'd have to watch Kelley's new, younger husband grabbing her ass at some violin recital. I would show up for our daughter's college graduation in a wheelchair, feebly waving with a purple-veined hand. Eventually I'd be stashed away in the nursing home, and our daughter would groan when another Sunday rolled around and her mother reminded her it was time to visit Papaw.

"Mom, he drools."

"I know, honey. But he loves you."

I was terrified that I would have a heart attack and not live to see this theoretical child grow up. However many years I had left, I could not see spending them as Kelley's junior partner. I didn't want any pit bulls in the house. I couldn't imagine changing diapers and lugging strollers through airports and sliding thermometers into a baby's ass at 5:00 a.m. I wanted to follow Springsteen on tour in Europe. I wanted to float in the pure blue waters off a Greek island.

I waited for a night when Nat and Sam were with their mother. When Kelley arrived, I told her we needed to talk. She heard the predictable words tumbling out of my mouth and told me to shut up.

"You're not breaking up with me," she said. "I'm breaking up with you."

She smiled with the weary expression of someone who had been rehearsing. She told me that I was a cheat and a liar and a pathetic excuse for a man. In slow motion she stood and headed for the door. There was almost nothing of hers to retrieve from the bedroom. Knowing this day was coming, she had been spiriting away her clothes for weeks, emptying the house of her traces. I'd been too self-absorbed to notice.

As she walked out, I held my breath again as though it were midnight and I were still driving past the frozen clock. Only now, I truly was dead.

Hurricane Katrina hit New Orleans the following Monday, and soon the news overran with images of corpses floating in dirty water.

I went into the newsroom and stared at my computer screen. Kelley's desk was empty for the next two weeks until she reappeared, possessed by a silent fury. When we passed near the elevators, she walked away as though I did not exist.

"Really?" I said. "This is what you want?"

The rituals of bitter dissolution played out for weeks. Seeking counsel, I went to Mike Wilson, our editor and mutual friend. Mike listened patiently as I asked if he could broker some kind of truce. He said he was sorry, but there was nothing he could do. The stalemate deepened. From across the room, I could see that Kelley was losing weight, buying flattering clothes, projecting an aura of triumphant defiance. She was smiling and laughing with her pod mates, all of them women who I thought were my friends but who were now avoiding eye contact.

I tried to distract myself with a trip to Target. It was late September now. Nat and Sam were still excited about our party, so I couldn't cancel it. When I arrived at the store, a fresh Halloween display awaited. I was walking among the gargoyles, admiring their snarling faces, when I stopped. I thought about the winged dog Kelley had given me. The Guardian of Hopes and Dreams. That was its fucking name.

I don't know how long I stood there, as other shoppers pushed their carts around me. A Target was the last place on earth to expect an epiphany, but the realizations came flooding.

I felt a stab as I remembered the daughter I'd wanted since I was a boy. Wasn't that one of the reasons I'd been drawn to Kelley? At our first dinner, long before the midnight drives began, hadn't I told her how much I wanted to cradle that child in my arms?

When I got home, I was sobbing, pacing, talking to myself. I literally could not stand up straight.

I sought out my old counselor, who had helped me through my divorce. In the weeks of marathon sessions that followed, she helped me untangle everything I'd gotten wrong. I told her what I wanted, and she asked if I was sure. Maybe I preferred to keep jumping from relationship to relationship, plotting escape routes.

One night I sat in my living room and opened my laptop. The mummies were already positioned before the big front window. Now they stood sentinel behind me, listening to my fingertips on the keyboard.

I wrote for hours, deleting and starting over and deleting again, trying to find the words to prove that for once my words meant something. I had no idea if it was too late.

At 2:44 a.m., I hit "send."

Kelley

The Gulf water lay flat and still, and November cold, and so pale as it stretched toward the sky that the horizon faded into rumor.

I'd grown up surrounded by it. I'd squelched my toes into its sandy floor, never wading farther than neck-deep. I'd swallowed bits of it trying to belly-surf its waves toward the shore. I'd dangled my fishhook into its murky expanse from the side of a boat. I had admired it only safely, distantly, the way people appreciate zoo animals and museum art.

Now I stood on the slick desk of the *Anastasi,* a forty-six-foot sponging boat, a relic of another time anchored off the coast of Tarpon Springs, Florida. I was reporting on a dying way of life. When I am reporting, I get to forget who I am. I was almost three months past the breakup, about a month past Tom's e-mail. I was adrift. I could stare off the boat in any direction and see nothing but water and sky.

"Mermaid," Tasso called to me.

He was sunbaked and ox-strong. If I'd wanted a hero to distract me from my troubles and ravage me in the salt spray, he could have played the part in a pinch. He was one of the last Greek sponge divers, wringing out a living on the ocean floor.

He had speared grouper through the eye and punched a shark in the nose.

Tasso believed the only way to know the sea was to sink into it, surrender to it. He wanted me to follow him down into the deep. Red tide was poisoning the ocean. He was searching for life in the water. I wasn't sure I was ready to admit it yet, but I was trying to salvage something, too.

I was as seaworthy as a giraffe. I certainly didn't know how to dive. Tasso slipped a mask over my face and hooked my fingers around his belt. "Mermaid," he said, "just hold on."

Down we went.

I was helpless, in another realm. So much heavy water above, so small a space inside that plastic mask. My breath came fast and loud, but then the fizz began to clear and I saw the sand, white on the floor, and the sponges swaying like alien life, and the fish, darting and shimmering, and Tasso, half swimming, half running against the current, as if nothing could stop him, as if he could part the sea. I was some forgotten piece of kelp, trailing him in the current. I was water. I was air. I was at the mercy of the waves and the sun, and oh my God, it was beautiful down there.

I stayed on the water with Tasso for four days. As the sky lightened in the mornings, I drank his Greek tea with honey while he shaved with salt water and a straight razor. All day he dove. He would rise out of the water and unzip his wetsuit and stone crab claws would rain out onto the deck. At night I drifted off in the salt breezes, rocked by the ocean. I thought about Tom, of course, because I missed him and I wanted to go to his door and tell him enough already and melt into his arms, but I had no phone, no computer, no Internet, and I had long ago realized that I could not change him or fix him. I surrendered to that, too.

It had taken me days to respond to his e-mail. By the time he'd sent it, my rage and disgust had corroded everything, and I didn't even want to read it. I had cried all I was willing to cry.

After the breakup, I'd spent a week in bed. Mike, my boss, would call to check on me, and I'd cry into the pillow, at times unable to form words. "I'm sorry, sugar," Mike would say. After making excuses for me as long as he could, he sent me to New Orleans in the aftermath of Katrina, and by the time I got back I had absorbed the fury of that storm. I was bent on destruction. All those lies. All those wasted years.

Mike never meddled. He just listened. "Are you feeling any better about Tom?" he asked one day in September. "God, no," I told him. "Last night I had a dream where I ran over him with my car."

I'd lost too much time at work, and too much dignity.

Then the e-mail came.

> i hope you'll find it in your heart to read this.

In it, I saw a broken and sorry man, and I guess there was satisfaction in that. But he was only looking inward at the mess he had made of his own life. He didn't acknowledge the carnage he had wrought in mine.

> i have never felt such a deep and crushing regret.
> i feel your absence every minute of every day.

Tasso's given name, Anastasios, and the name of his boat, *Anastasi,* both meant the same thing: resurrected. We were all looking for new life. By the time I got back to shore, I knew I was going to have that life, and a baby and a dog and a goddamned picket fence, with Tom or without him. I would be okay. I was good at rescuing things, but you can fight against the current for only so long before it sweeps you away. Tom would have to save himself.

I had written Tom back and agreed to meet with him, but only after he completed a gauntlet of conditions. He probably answered various riddles and made certain offerings before the gods. I demanded counseling: mine, his, and ours. I grilled and berated him in my counselor's office and refused to see him without a referee. We ended up, eventually, in the office of a couples counselor neither of us had ever met. Neutral territory.

"How long have you been married?" she asked.

"Oh no, we are not married," I told her. "We are not even dating."

She startled in her chair. This was not something she saw every day.

"Are you here to get together," she asked, "or to split for good?"

That question cut through my defenses. I could humiliate Tom without her ninety-dollar-an-hour assistance. I was there, I had to admit, because I wanted everything he was saying to be true.

I don't know how we edged our way back. I remember that it took a long time, that he was as broken and humbled a person as I'd ever seen. I didn't attend his stupid Halloween party, and I asked a friend to check his dresser drawers to make sure I had gotten all my stuff. Part of me never wanted to see that house again.

While I wrote the story of Tasso and the sponge boat, Tom was working on a big series for the paper. Both of us wrote late into the night, alone in our dark corners of the newsroom, not speaking, stealing glances at each other between paragraphs. Late one night, I messaged him a compliment on his story, and he messaged back, and pretty soon I was leaving my laptop open all the time, in case.

He would tell me he loved me, and I wouldn't respond. I had seen him in counseling a few times, but I wasn't ready to talk in person or on the phone. I didn't allow myself to dwell on his promise to commit. It would be cruel to want that again and lose it, again. I hated him and loved him, and my only shelter was distance—the buffer of the newsroom, the protective shield of the computer screen. It all fell apart when we ended up, by coincidence, at the same conference in Boston.

Tom was scheduled to give a reading in a large auditorium in front of a thousand people. I made a friend sit next to me and scrunched in my chair, trying to meld into the crowd. I hoped he couldn't see me.

He stood at the lectern in a suit. He cleared his throat.

This is a love story like no other, he began. *Boy meets girl.*

My cheeks caught fire. I grabbed my friend by the arm.

Girl decides that boy is wrong, all wrong, and that the forces of darkness have possibly replaced him with a copy of the original...

He was reading to me. The story was one he had written years earlier, about two people brought together by forces beyond their understanding.

In that moment, the questions of Laura's life—questions that would run through all the years stretching before her—announced themselves once and for all. Was it brave of her to venture out into the hurricane? Or was it foolish?

Tom, like the character in his story, had stepped inside a storm. He was drenched in it. I could destroy him. Maybe I already had. He had been ruled by fear for so long it had warped and twisted him into a dark copy of himself. He was turning into the wind, letting the rain hammer and shape him into something new.

She felt the ecstasy surging inside her. She turned her face to the dark skies, surrendering to the power and grace and glory of things beyond her control.

That night we talked, sitting close in the hotel bar, stone sober.

We sat next to each other on the plane home.

A few days before Christmas, I let him come over. I had spent four days putting lights on the tree. We sat on the couch and talked, and it grew late, and I couldn't ask him to stay and I couldn't ask him to leave, so we just stayed on that couch all night, barely moving, sharing space and air. He kissed my forehead, and I turned, a little.

The next night I threw a futon mattress in front of the fireplace, and we slept on it in the shimmer of a thousand lights.

Ten months later, I was walking down the aisle, holding Nat by the arm. Mike, the best man either of us would ever know, stood next to Tom, holding the ring.

Tom

Another morning in the kingdom of thwarted creation. Bright blue skies outside, a mist of palpable aching in the waiting room within. In the hushed silence, women gathered themselves and stared into the distance, opening their purses, closing them, opening them again. I sat off to the side, on a couch so soft and deep that its embrace nearly swallowed me. I tried to render myself invisible. I had my own anxieties to manage.

Unsure of where to direct my gaze, I studied the room's orchestrated serenity. The walls hung with paintings of blue and pink flowers, perpetually blooming. Deep green sofas and deep green carpet, dark wood tables, the entrance adorned with ferns. All of it suggested a spring meadow surrounded by forest. Had Sherwin-Williams created a palette just for fertility clinics?

From the moment of my epiphany in the Target, I had never wavered in my desire to have a baby with Kelley. More than two years had gone by, and we had lost track of how many doctors we'd seen. Nothing was working. Kelley was thirty-four now, and I was fifty-one. All the time I'd squandered had delayed us too long.

"Thomas French?"

Guilty! I mean…

"Yes."

A nurse led me into the labyrinth of yearning, past wall charts ripe with cross-sectioned drawings of ovaries and Fallopian tubes, past posters brimming with blastocysts and zygotes, past exam room after exam room where I had held Kelley's hand. Finally, we arrived at the only room reserved for patients with Y chromosomes. The door was marked with what appeared to be a cartoonish icon of a smiling sperm similar to the happy teeth that cavort on the walls at the dentist's office. I stepped inside, blinking. Were my nerves playing tricks? Had I imagined the dancing sperm?

I turned to look again at the door, but the nurse was already shutting it behind us. She handed me a sheet of instructions and an empty plastic cup.

"Wash your hands thoroughly first," she said, avoiding eye contact. "When you're done, leave the cup on the sink."

Then she was gone, leaving me in the Room of Requirement. A black faux-leather recliner awaited, along with a pile of girlie magazines, a couple of DVDs of porn, and a DVD player and TV. I was already embarrassed and irritated. Now the shabbiness of these props nudged me toward outrage. If the rest of the clinic was defined by every cliché of feminine aesthetics, this room had been designed as a shrine to the assumption that men are essentially farm animals, devoid of subtlety or difference, that our sexual response is so predictable that a few visual cues are all any of us need, at any place and at any time. My resentment was compounded by the fact that most of the men I knew, including myself, proved those assumptions true every day.

I turned to the instructions. I was to fill out a label on the cup with my name and date of birth. I was to be careful not to let either my fingers or any other appendage touch the interior of the cup. I stopped at a warning against engaging in any oral contact to encourage an erection, because saliva might contaminate the sample. This stumped me. I was alone; in fact, the clinic's rules forbade wives and girlfriends from joining their men in this room. Was oral contact even possible? Were any men that limber?

I was to do my best, the sheet said, to keep the sample inside the cup. The hectoring tone made it clear that the people in charge had no confidence that the Neanderthals in this room would be willing or able to control the path of their DNA. I looked around, wishing for a hazmat suit. Surely they brought in a black light and a pressure hose now and then. The cup itself was big enough to accommodate the output of a rhinoceros. Did they expect me to fill that?

Enough whining, I told myself, remembering everything Kelley had gone through. The consultations and the ultra-sounds, the speculums and catheters, including one that the nurses dubbed the Tomcat. If she had endured all of that, I could face the task before me now.

The magazines were not tempting. Some *Penthouses*, a few sorry issues of *Hustler,* all several years old, all obviously having been thumbed through countless times. The DVDs held no allure. The only title I saw—*Ass Masters Volume 16,* something like that—confused me. A man walks in here, trying to help his wife make a baby, and you encourage him to fantasize about sodomizing surgically enhanced porn stars? The bulletin board down the hall showed snapshots of dozens of infants and toddlers conceived, presumably, with the assistance of *Ass Masters 16*. Who was I to judge? If Kelley thought it would guarantee her pregnancy, she would have gift-wrapped me the first fifteen volumes.

Time was slipping away, faster and faster. I still remembered the teenage girl I'd met at the writers' camp, with the spiral perm and the shy smile. If anyone had told me that we'd end up together, I would never have believed it. She was so young. So serious. Sixteen years later, she'd walked down the aisle like a luminous dream.

After moving in with me and the boys, Kelley had quickly taken over. She left Huck to stay with her mother but had already begun turning our garage into a nursery for hordes of foster puppies. One day, watching Kelley pull six newborns from their birth sacs, Sam had nearly fainted. Before I knew it, I was walking pit bulls through the neighborhood. Kelley had been right; they were easily the friendliest breed. They loved climbing into our laps, even though they were far too big. The only foster dog that had attacked me was a little dachshund mother who clamped onto the bottom of my shorts one day when I strayed too close to her newborns. I told her it was all right, that I would never hurt her babies, and she'd waddled away, growling. One day, surfing Petfinder, Kelley had spotted a beautiful brown-and-white pit-bull mix who was slated to be put down that day. Kelley had a feeling about this dog and made a couple of calls to have her spared. Soon we were adopting her, and we named her Muppet. My boys and I serenaded this dog with silly songs.

> I try really hard to do nobody harm
> I can't help if I'm lick-y, it's part of my charm...

Kelley's transformation of our family was well under way. That summer, when the seventh and final installment of *Harry Potter* went on sale at midnight, she herded us to the nearest Walmart to wait together in a line that stretched through women's lingerie.

I was no longer a reporter at the *St. Pete Times*. After working there for twenty-seven years, I had accepted a buyout and taken a teaching job on the journalism faculty at Indiana University, my alma mater. Kelley had a fulfilling job as an editor in St. Pete, and she wasn't ready to move. Now I was commuting every week, flying to Indiana on Tuesday nights and flying back to Florida a couple of days later. It was stressful, but it worked.

After more than a year of therapy, I had made my peace with the fear of being too old to become a father again. My grandmother had lived into her nineties. My dad was approaching eighty and going strong.

"Nobody knows how much time they have," Kelley told me. "Your genes are good."

Time to stop procrastinating. Trying to drown out the voices passing back and forth in the corridor outside, I settled into the recliner, unzipped my jeans, and put aside my complaints about the objectification of men objectifying women. I was just another Neanderthal. Just a man, no better or worse than any other.

The results came back a few days later. My sperm count was somewhere above eighty million. They were energetic and fast and swam straight.

The numbers floored me. Eighty million versions of me, wriggling toward one of Kelley's eggs. I had interviewed an embryologist once, and he'd explained how the sperm gathered outside the zona pellucida, a layer of glycoproteins encasing the egg. *Zona pellucida.* I loved the way the words rolled off the tongue. The embryologist had spoken with great passion about the science of in vitro fertilization, where eggs are paired with sperm inside petri dishes and allowed to fertilize outside the woman's body. But he had also spoken with reverence about the mysteries of creation. Over his incubator, he had hung a poster from Michelangelo's painting on the ceiling of the Sistine Chapel. The close-up showed God and Adam reaching toward each other as a spark of life arced between their fingertips.

Eighty million possibilities. All those variations, all those different futures.

The sense of wonder had been easy to hold on to at first. Then time began to tick away in twenty-eight-day cycles. We tried to laugh about it, make light of the pressure, lose ourselves in the simplicity of desire. But every month Kelley grew more disappointed, and I grew more certain that God was punishing me and penalizing Kelley for putting up with me. For all my genuine remorse, my sins were not so easily washed away.

More doctors, more encounters with the Tomcat. I held her hand, again and again, as they probed her, first with a nine-inch transvaginal wand that she called the Dick of Death and later with a mini–video camera that snaked through her navel to map her inner landscape.

"Here," the doctor told me afterward, pointing to something fuzzy on the screen. "Those are her ovaries. There's her uterus..."

When it was time for the first round of IVF, we drove together to the clinic in Tampa. I had read that a man's output increased the longer he stayed aroused, so I begged her to help. We had a good forty-five-minute drive to the clinic. Why waste it?

"Come on," I said. "Can't you just talk dirty a little?"

Kelley sighed the sigh of a woman who had already suffered deeper indignities. She hopped into the backseat and started to whisper into my ear. Real or feigned, her performance was all I needed. We maintained the charade all the way through St. Petersburg, across the glittering expanse of Tampa Bay, through morning rush hour in downtown Tampa. Out of the corner of my eye, I could see truck drivers in the next lane, staring down from their cabs at our windows, grinning.

By the time we pulled into the clinic parking lot, we were both laughing. Five days later, the doctors gave us a black-and-white photo that showed the two blastocysts we'd created, floating side by side, their cells already dividing in the darkness.

We knew the odds were not high for either embryo to survive long enough to become a fetus. Even so we were hopeful until Kelley started taking pregnancy tests, and tossing them into the trash. By now we had spent more than $20,000 on fertility treatments. Kelley didn't think the money mattered. To her, our daughter was already a real person.

"What if someone took Nat or Sam from you?" she asked one day in bed. "What would you pay to get them back?"

The toll of so many dashed hopes was showing. We were lashing out at each other, hearing judgment and recrimination where none was intended, fighting over nothing. Every day I could see the sadness clouding Kelley's face. I saw it when she came home from work and slumped against the kitchen counter. She was drowning in disappointment.

Several months later, we tried another round. This time, the doctors told us that three embryos had survived in their petri dishes. As was common in IVF clinics around the United States, our team had ethical protocols that encouraged them to place a maximum of two embryos inside a womb. Nobody wanted another Octomom. Their plan was to put two into Kelley and to freeze the third for later.

The embryo transfer was scheduled for a Sunday morning. Kelley was stretched out on the table, in her gown and ready to go, when she informed the team that in fact they were going to put all three embryos inside her. I watched, in awe, as she ordered one of the nurses to call the clinic's head doctor at home and ask her to override the protocols.

"I want those babies inside me," Kelley said. "I'm not leaving a man behind."

I would have killed to hear exactly what the doctor said when she got that call, to know whether she was laughing or sighing. But when the nurse hung up, she said they had permission to go forward. The team scattered to make their final prep for putting three embryos inside the crazy woman. They put a piece of paper in front of us, asking us to confirm that we understood that triplets were possible. Kelley signed without a glance.

I stood over my wife, admiring her ruthlessness.

"Triplets?" I said, laughing.

"We'll be fine," she said.

The chances were small that any of the three embryos would make it. A couple of weeks later, a blood test confirmed what we already knew.

Kelley

People say that engineering a child in a lab separates creation from an act of love, but people say lots of stupid things.

Babies are created from all manner of impulses. They are created in the backseats of cars, in bathroom stalls, up against alley walls, under bleachers, and in stairwells. They come from desire, lust, confusion, capitulation, revenge, even rage.

Babies built in labs are the product of meticulous calculation. They come only at great cost—second jobs and second mortgages. They are built by committee. There are so many opportunities to turn back.

I've heard people call fertility treatment selfish, and that has never made sense. Children hijack your body, your money, your time, your privacy, your very identity. IVF is excellent preparation for parenthood, because the driving question at every turn is *How much can you give?*

First it's just a few tests, maybe some pills, and there are headaches and mood swings, and then a simple procedure, some mild cramping, a day or two off work, then let's try this minor surgery, and pretty soon a box of needles and vials arrives in the mail and your fridge looks like a pharmacy and you're in the middle of a science experiment and you don't know how you got there. "Why don't you just adopt?" everyone asks, as if that were as simple as stopping by the orphanage on the way home from work. Adoption can be at least as costly and daunting as IVF, and few couples have the resources to pursue both at once.

Now we were four years in. The doctors wanted us to consider using eggs from a donor. Donor eggs are something of a magic bullet in infertility treatment, the way swapping out the entire engine will solve car trouble. Doctors can make a baby with just one sperm. The egg is far more mysterious and more difficult to obtain.

After giving up so much already, severing my genetic link to my child came without a twinge. I don't presume that my genes are so precious. My stepsons don't carry them, and they are magnificent. My three older siblings were born from a different mother. We look nothing alike. We speak with different accents. So what.

I'm proud of the work ethic I inherited from my parents and grandparents. My mother and her mother both worked into their seventies. But I don't need biology to pass along their example. I'm proud of my mother's selflessness. When she married my dad, she got three stepkids, ages eight, ten, and twelve. Then, five months later, she got me. She drove a 1964 Ford Falcon and wore my Plumb Elementary School T-shirts until I went to college. Her hands were forever rough from the chemicals at the hospital lab where she worked, but they always felt good to me. I could pass on the best parts of her by my example, and without the bunions.

We don't yet understand all the ways biology shapes us. But having a child was not about creating someone in my own image. I wanted to help my daughter become the best version of herself, not another me. I had an image in my head, sure, of a dark-haired, blue-eyed, dirty-faced girl. But I hoped she would surprise me and challenge me. The real gift of creation is the thing that no one has ever seen before.

"You know," Tom told me one day in the car, "if you have a daughter, she'll grow up to be a teenager who hates you, for a while."

"It's not her job to love me," I said finally. "It's my job to love her. That's it."

I owed her an amazing father. I owed her my complete devotion and my best effort at a good example. I owed her the best genes I could find. She owed me nothing.

But who was the woman walking around with the germ of my daughter in her belly? The anonymous-donor route never made sense to me. My daughter was going to want answers. I owed her that, too.

Tom and I scrolled through websites of potential donors provided by agencies that specialized in these things. Page after page of pretty women, mostly white, most no older than twenty-five, all, it seemed, hoping to subsidize their education. Nursing, accounting, and teaching were popular choices. They said they wanted to help a couple in need bring life into the world, and yes, they could really use the cash. They supplied photos of themselves in swimsuits and evening wear. They posted baby pictures. Allergy profiles. Medical histories. This one liked walks on the beach and competitive running. That one was allergic to shellfish and cats. This one's eggs cost $5,000. That one had produced children before, so hers cost $8,000.

Nothing in those online profiles told me what I needed to know. Did they have a sense of humor? Were they creative? Were they brave? Were they strong?

Tom would barely look at the websites. He was in an impossible spot. Choosing a donor meant conceding that he found her attractive, and given the impending masturbatory act, well. He pretty much let me handle things.

"Whose eggs would you want?" he asked me one day. "If you could have any eggs in the world?"

Tom was always asking me strange, deep questions, then getting annoyed when I went silent for twenty minutes while considering my response. But I answered this one in a blink.

"Jennifer's."

She was my secret crush. My friend's wife. Gorgeous, funny, sarcastic, she was intoxicating to me in every way. But I barely knew her, and anyway, I would never ask anyone for a favor so huge. I had admired her at parties as I fumbled through small talk. She was one of those women who stumbled out of bed every morning ready to film a shampoo commercial. I swear, she glowed. Whenever I was around her, I felt like I had three heads.

I knew her husband better. Ben was a reporter who worked for me at the paper, though it was hard for me to consider myself his boss. He did his thing, and I helped however I could. Sometimes that meant bringing him a midnight burrito while he wrote toward dawn; once it meant putting a plane ticket on my credit card so he could get out of Haiti. I always felt like I learned more from him than he did from me.

One day at work, I summoned Ben to my cubicle.

"Check this out," I said, turning my monitor so he could peruse the donor profiles in all their glossy-haired glory. "I'm shopping for a baby mama."

"Whaaat?"

Straight hair, curly hair, freckles, cheekbones, melanoma, long legs, depression, Alzheimer's, breast cancer, dark lashes, thigh gap, green eyes, cholesterol. All there in the menu, like ordering a sub from Jimmy John's. Everything was a choice. Someday, I'd explain to my daughter why she burned instead of tanned, or why her boobs were so big or so small, or why she got cavities even though she flossed.

"It's weird, right?" I said. "I mean, could I even stand to be in a room with any of these people?"

Ben didn't know about my crush on his wife and her ripe, golden eggs. I knew he understood what I was talking about. He was all about the intangibles, and he'd built a family that cared about character, not pedigree. His three kids were always naked in their yard, singing or climbing or collecting bugs, falling off the roof of the shed. They protested injustices on street corners with homemade signs. They testified before the county commission. They were raised to think for themselves, to give a damn, and to wring the world for all its joy.

Jennifer always had a beer in one hand and a baby on the hip. She was every bit as gifted as her husband. Her Twitter account was warped domestic poetry.

> Got Bey to eat an olive today by telling him it was an eyeball. Not sure what that says about him, or me.

> Are lost-cat signs necessary? Isn't it just a less direct way of telling everyone your cat is dead?

> A teacher just told me she needed die-cut letters. I smiled and nodded. Now I'm scared and alone and confused. Where am I? #PTA

Some weeks later Jennifer and I ended up together in the back of a New York City taxicab. Ben had won a big journalism award, and we were on our way to a dinner to pick up a plaque. Jennifer was sitting beside me, looking like she'd just pulled something out of the dryer and run her fingers through her hair and was now totally going to dominate these journalism nerds, when she turned to me and said, "You can have my eggs."

I couldn't speak, of course. She didn't know what she was talking about, obviously. What the hell did Ben say to her, anyway? I couldn't feel my face.

"We should drink, a lot, and then talk about this," I said finally.

We arrived at the Mexican restaurant where all the reporters and editors and contest administrators were making small talk and congratulating one another, and Jennifer and I drank pomegranate margaritas and huddled and whispered about egg stimulation, progesterone shots, and what if the baby likes you better than me. It was the longest conversation I'd ever had with her, and it continued all the way back to Florida, through e-mails and texts and dinners and doctor appointments. If she ever wavered, it didn't show. Our family trees were branching in directions that nature never anticipated. If this worked, we would be linked forever. Our kids would be half siblings, sort of. Egg siblings?

Eventually Ben and I sat down with Mike. We wanted to be up-front with him, because the work element complicated things, and because he was our friend. I was nervous, and Mike could tell it was serious, and it occurred to me that he probably thought Ben and I were having an affair.

"Ben and I," I started, hesitantly, "and Tom and Jennifer," I continued, studying his face, "are going to make a baby," I said. "Together."

Mike started to cry.

Other people would think it was weird, but who cared? We didn't have all the answers, but I believed we'd figure them out.

It was a crazy way to make a baby, I guess. But if there was not love in it, then I don't know what love is, or what it's for.

Tom

My wife didn't try to hide the fact that she was falling for someone else. I would see her flirting on the phone, and I would know
that Jennifer was on the other end. They texted each other in the
dead time after lunch and whispered together late at night. Like
so many newly infatuated couples, they shared their secret selves
in a running conversation that filled the in-between spaces of
their lives. Afterward, Kelley would sit, openly besotted, and
stare into space. If I tried to approach while she was still in the
afterglow, she would ignore me. Then she would snap out of it
and gush about how clever and brilliant Jennifer was, how
funny, how gorgeous.

"I mean, she's unbelievably hot. Don't you think so?"

I knew not to agree too emphatically. I would admit that,
yes, Jennifer was beautiful, but then I would add that Kelley was
beautiful, too. I would point out how they both had long flowing hair, how the bone structure of their faces was similar, how
they easily could be mistaken for sisters.

"No," Kelley would say, waving me off. "Jennifer is in a
whole different category of hotness."

Nothing would be gained from pressing my point. Jennifer
had an edgy, magnetic charm. On Facebook, she referred to her
home as House of the Tragically Hip, and no one gave her a

hard time about it, because it was true. When her son Bey gave her a Mother's Day card, he said she was as pretty as Mexico, and as sweet as dandelions, and as smart as Iron Man. She told people that she was brainwashing her children to be kind and openhearted. Whenever possible, she railed against racists and ideologues and violent cops.

"What do we do when we see the police?" she asked her kids.

"Film them," they said.

I was thrilled that Kelley was so happy with her choice. Together, she and Jennifer were going to make a baby. At some point, I would be summoned to make my contribution, but something different was happening between the two of them. Something fairly new in human history. One woman's egg, another woman's womb, one man's sperm. If we ended up with a child, Jennifer's chromosomes and mine would be intertwined in every cell of that child's body. We would be joined in the most profound and lasting act of creation, and yet we would never do more than hug. The real bond, the one that mattered, was blossoming between these two women.

Like Kelley, I had heard all the windy denunciations of IVF, the grim reminders of the test-tube babies colonized for servitude in *Brave New World*. Children born from IVF had even been labeled Frankenstein babies. The naysayers had ignored a fundamental distinction. Mary Shelley's monster had been resurrected from the dead. IVF opened a path for the creation of an entirely new life. How exactly did these babies' time inside a petri dish turn them into monsters? Perhaps they had been denied a divine light.

I had no moral qualms about how far Kelley and I were going in order to make a child. But there was no denying that we were tinkering with the most essential mechanics of human experience. The nuns in my head reminded me that the Catholic Church had always decreed IVF to be a sin. Searching Church doctrine on the web, I learned that the crux of the objections involved the detour from the usual path—the way IVF babies are engineered in clinics as opposed to being created from an act of love between husband and wife. The Church was even more harsh on the use of egg and sperm donors, because this meant that half of the child's genetic material would originate from someone outside the bounds of marriage. The deepest outrage was reserved for the question of what happens to embryos that are left over and are either discarded or frozen or donated to other couples, or sometimes used in research.

The essence of the Church's objections was that IVF put parents in the position of making decisions better left to God. All of it, the Church said, was violence committed against the dignity of human life.

"Inherent in IVF," one site proclaimed, "is the treatment of children, in their very coming into being, as less than human beings."

My imaginary nuns clucked righteously over this last point. But it was hard for me to take such warnings too seriously, coming as they did from an institution that had allowed its priests to molest and rape thousands of children and then did its best to hide these offenses.

The Church raised important questions about what happens to the embryos that don't grow into babies. Kelley and I had signed paperwork stipulating that if we ever did end up with extra embryos, we would pay to have them frozen for us to use later.

Before the egg donation with Jennifer could go forward, the clinic required that we all meet with a counselor who specialized in fertility issues. Jennifer and Ben went in first while Kelley and I had coffee across the street. Then Kelley and I went in while Jennifer and Ben stepped out. Then the counselor talked to all four of us at once.

She asked Jennifer if she would feel conflicted once the baby was born. Would she harbor any claim? Jennifer said she was very clear that this was going to be Kelley's baby, not hers. She pointed out that she already had three children of her own.

The counselor asked all of us whether we planned to keep the egg donation a secret from our families and friends. Ben and Jennifer were already talking with their children about what was happening. I also believed it was best not to keep this secret, but Kelley wanted to take some time to think before announcing the baby's parentage. It was the baby's business, she reasoned. It was deeply personal information that perhaps should not be broadcast without her consent.

The counselor wanted to know if Kelley and I had thought through what to tell our child. Would we want the baby to meet Jennifer and Ben and their kids? Yes.

Egg donation was still new enough, the counselor said, that there wasn't much research yet into the emotional effects of such decisions. But studies seemed to show that children did better when their parents opened up with them early on.

The counselor turned to Kelley.

"What happens if something goes wrong with your pregnancy or if the baby is born with some kind of genetic problem? Will you be angry with Jennifer for giving you a defective egg?"

Kelley said she was still stunned that Jennifer and Ben had volunteered such a gift. She was sure that the only things she would ever feel toward them were love and gratitude, no matter what.

In the middle of this, Kelley and I took Sam to Pittsburgh to start his freshman year at Carnegie Mellon. It had been hard taking Nat to college three years before. But this was much more painful, since Sam's departure left our lives unbearably quiet. When Sam wasn't looking, I wrote one of our favorite quotes on a little eraser board that hung on the door of his dorm room. It was from the first pages of Cormac McCarthy's *The Road.*

He knew only that the child was his warrant. He said: If he is not the word of God God never spoke.

When we hugged Sam good-bye, all three of us were shaking. I cried for hours. I had always been at my best with my sons, and now they were gone. Without them, I didn't know who I was.

Kelley held me for the rest of that night as I babbled on and on.

"I don't want to walk into that house and see his room so empty. I just can't take it. We have to have another baby. We have to make all this fertility stuff work. I need a little baby to hold."

Kelley smiled and pulled me close.

"We're working on it, sugar."

The hormone treatments began two months later, with both Kelley and Jennifer receiving daily injections to sync their cycles.

Early one morning, I arrived at the hospital and found Jennifer lying in one of the rooms in her gown, waiting to be prepped for the egg retrieval. Ben and Kelley had both been delayed, and for a few awkward minutes, it was just me sitting alone beside this extraordinary woman who was giving us something irreplaceable. A new life. A future. I wanted to tell her how much it meant, but I was too choked up, so I patted her arm and asked if she was okay and tried to make small talk until it was time for the doctors to roll her away.

A nurse led me to another Room of Requirement. Somewhere else in the hospital, the doctors removed eight eggs from Jennifer. Ben and Kelley had arrived by then, and when Jennifer was released, the three of us rolled her in a wheelchair toward the parking lot. Jennifer was still groggy. Ben was so focused on making sure that she was all right that he walked straight into a wall and smashed the cup of coffee in his hand, spraying all of us in warm droplets. We laughed, but already Kelley and I were wondering what the embryologist was doing right at that moment. Had he already injected the sperm into the petri dishes? Had he put them into the incubator? How long would it take the first swimmer to reach one of the eggs and for the cell to begin dividing in that limbo of darkness?

Five days later, a nurse brought us photos of our four embryos and pointed to the two that the doctor had chosen to transfer to Kelley's womb. They looked like oatmeal cookies.

When the doctor used a catheter to insert the embryos, I held Kelley's hand as I had held it through so many other procedures. Maybe that's what being a husband was really about. Not paying the bills or taking out the trash or even making love. Maybe it was just about holding your wife's hand.

A week and a half later, I woke up in the night and heard

Kelley stirring. She went to the bathroom, and when she came back I gave her a look.

"I just know we're going to have a baby," I told her.

"I know," she said.

"I mean it," I said. "It's going to happen, sweetheart."

"I know," she said.

I caught something in her voice. She wasn't just appeasing me so I'd let her go back to sleep.

"Why do you feel so much more confident this time?" I asked.

She drew close and wrapped her arms around me and whispered into my ear.

"Two positive pregnancy tests."

I sat up. I was having trouble processing what she was saying.

"Wait..."

PART TWO

Blood

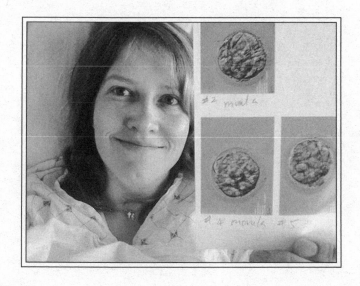

Kelley

Our baby came swirling into view, week after week, on the grainy wedge of the ultrasound monitor. First a dark featureless pool, then a tiny orb, then budding arms and legs and finally long fingers and a recognizable profile. Everything had been so hard. Now the promise of our child unfolded easily.

I tracked the baby's growth with an iPhone app. When we told Nat and Sam, their future sibling was the size of a sesame seed. Then a blueberry. Then an orange. Why was the metaphor always produce? I scrubbed the baseboards in the spare bedroom and stopped buttoning my jeans. Tom and I couldn't agree on a name, but we made endless lists. I texted every ultrasound to Jennifer, who texted back her appraisal.

> Jennifer: If what I think are its fingers are actually its fingers, aren't they big? Do you think the baby will have giant fingers?
> Me: I think they look like claws. Like a T. rex.
> Jennifer: That would be cool.

At week twelve, the fertility doctor handed me off to my regular ob-gyn, the assured and handsome Dr. McNeill, and his adorably dimpled partner, Dr. Reyes. I scrutinized those ultrasounds. I asked a million questions.

At around week sixteen, I went in to learn the baby's gender. Tom was at work in Indiana, and I was used to going to appointments alone. I was used to the cold ultrasound gel on my belly and even the Dick of Death. They could do whatever they wanted to me now.

"What are you hoping for?" the tech asked. I didn't want to say. As much as I loved Nat and Sam, I was ready for estrogen in the house.

The tech started searching, and when she got close, soon even I saw it. The world's biggest baby penis.

"Definitely a boy," the tech said.

Disappointment must have swept my face, though I tried not to feel it.

Pokemon. Circumcision (?). *Yu-Gi-Oh! Grand Theft Auto.* Beyblades. Poker. Wrestling. Ball scratching. Zombie movies. Street gangs.

"Wait," the tech said. She was still looking, slower now.

"I might have been wrong, but I can't tell. The baby's closing its legs."

She said I might have to come back. It might have been a baby penis, or it might have been the umbilical cord.

"I really need to know," I said. "I am going to wait it out."

More gel. Ticktock. Ticktock. The next patient getting antsy in the waiting room. Ticktock.

"There it is," she said. "Definitely a girl."

I sat upright on the table, laughing. "Are you sure?"

"Definitely."

Not long after, precisely on schedule, I felt her squirm and thump. She was like a pocket pet I carried everywhere. I loved talking to her, making plans. Tom was still gone three days a week, but I was never alone.

It felt as though Tom and I had, at last, gotten on track, but that wasn't entirely true. We were still two very different people, settled in our ways, chafing at the challenges of combining our lives. The joint checking account. The thermostat. The wounds we'd inflicted on each other in the early years as we lured each other close, then chased each other off. He stashed receipts and spare change behind books on the shelves, like a squirrel. I scurried after him, putting things in folders. He closed kitchen cabinets I'd left open and searched in vain for those little bread-bag tabs that I always threw out. I spent weekends battling the kudzu and neglect in the yard. He'd join me for a few minutes, then ask, "Can I have an inside chore?"

He disdained the boring details of real life, preferring to lose himself in stories of all kinds—books, movies, music. I wondered if he was avoiding me or if he was just avoiding everything. In the car, his music would be so loud we couldn't hear each other talk.

"Why are you so quiet?" he'd say.

"What?"

"Why are you looking at me like that?"

"What?!"

"Don't look at me like that!"

"I'm not!"

The baby reminded us that none of it mattered. Tom would put his face on my belly and sing to her—"Waitin' On a Sunny

Day," because we had waited so long, and it was starting to feel, finally, like the clouds were parting.

He wanted me to relax, but I never could. After work I scraped and repainted the doors and windowsills. I painted the baby's room, spackling and sanding every nail hole and scuff, erasing musk of teenage boy, smoothing on creamy layers of Water Chestnut in even strokes. I anchored the bookshelves to the wall studs. I hauled in a futon, a rocker, and a rug with a monkey on it. I would sit in the rocker and take it all in, the bright Matisse on the wall, the crisp trim. I'd contemplate the missing elements: the crib, the dresser, the baby. I knew all the ways we could still lose her. Tom urged me to take it easy on the decorating, we had plenty of time, but I pushed ahead. We had come too far.

On a Friday when I was around eighteen weeks pregnant, I put Muppet on a leash and took her for a bike ride after work. It was March, one of the rare pleasant Florida days before the oppressive humidity of summer settles in for good. Tom scolded me as I headed out the door — "Are you sure you want to take the dog? Why are you doing this?" — but I brushed him off. His caution was stifling.

As I pulled the bike out of the garage, I wondered how our divergent views on personal safety would play out in our parenting. I'd be taking the little tot out on her tricycle, and he'd come running after us, arms full of safety gear. He'd already unilaterally banned football and trampolines. Nat and Sam had never owned a dog or operated a power tool until I had come along. I wanted our child to grow up confident and unafraid. I had always been a shy kid. I wanted to raise a leader and a thinker. If she kept hearing *Be careful! Stop! Put that down!* I worried that she would learn not to trust herself.

I stayed on Woodlawn Circle, our wide, sun-dappled street, coasting downhill with Muppet trotting beside me. The street was lined with live oaks, and there was no traffic, but I scanned both sides for loose dogs or idiot neighbors. One woman, who hated pit bulls, liked to carry a baseball bat and spew threats at us. Muppet was half border collie, but I celebrated the pit-bull half, which I considered superior. Every time I passed the crazy woman's house, I imagined confrontations with her—sometimes verbal, sometimes criminal. Muppet had taken classes in obedience and agility and competed in a dog sport called flyball. She had an honest-to-God Canine Good Citizen certificate from the American Kennel Club. I imagined how well behaved Muppet would be in court, how she would impress the judge with her calm demeanor and polite handshake. Dozens of trainers from the local dog club would testify on her behalf. The crazy woman would be held in contempt.

At the halfway point, I clicked into a higher gear to let Muppet run. She loped happily, tongue lolling. Heading into the last quarter-mile, I slowed and downshifted, and out of nowhere came a snarling, bat-shit blur of fur. It couldn't have weighed more than five pounds, just cotton candy and teeth. Muppet veered sharply into the bike to get away, but the thing was on her. I was afraid if I dropped the leash, Muppet might have to defend herself, but because of her breed and size, she'd be whisked away by animal control no matter the provocation. Both dogs were in my spokes, and the bike was going down, and here came the little dog's owner, running into the street, and the bike toppled slowly, because we were barely moving anyway, and I landed on my knee. The dogs were both fine.

My jeans were ripped and my knee was bleeding, so Tom knew as soon as I walked in the door. I told him I was fine. His worry and disapproval hung in the air. I felt like a jerk. If anything happened to this baby, I'd have no one to blame but myself.

Two weeks later, at the twenty-week anatomy scan, the doctors checked every inch of the baby inside me, looking at her brain for excess fluid, at her face for a cleft palate or for a nasal structure that would indicate Down syndrome. Her spine, both in length and in cross section, showed no evidence of spina bifida. Her abdominal wall was closed, her diaphragm intact, intestines tucked neatly inside. Her heart had the right number of chambers, in the correct proportion, the valves opening and closing properly, 150 times per minute. The length of her femur, the circumference of her head and abdomen, all measured within normal ranges. That was a Friday.

On Sunday, I took Muppet to a flyball tournament. She was part of a dog racing team, the Tampa Bay Barkaneers, which sounds strange because it was. Four-dog teams raced each other carrying a ball over hurdles, sometimes trash-barking at each other across the lanes. People came from all over the state in RVs and SUVs, with packs of dogs bred for this purpose — mostly lithe border collies and spry Jack Russell terriers. It was a comic spectacle, like the obedience ring in *Best in Show*. One team's humans routinely pounded the mat and screamed, intentionally causing false starts to tire out the opponents' dogs. Tom rarely came to watch, and I didn't blame him.

Muppet would line up in the starting position, and I'd crouch next to her and whisper "Ready..." and her ears would flatten and her body would tense. "Set..." and she'd shift her weight to her back legs, frozen in anticipation. "Go." She'd fly down the lane, snatch a tennis ball from a ball launcher, kick-turn like a swimmer, and race back, 102 feet in 4.2 seconds. She never dropped the ball, swerved out of her lane, or missed a jump. She was rapidly collecting ribbons and titles, not that she knew, or cared. She was basted in the endorphins, the primitive part of her brain pinging *ball ball ball ball ball ball ball.* During one of the morning races, she came zipping back across the finish line and leapt at me for a celebratory hug and *wham,* nailed me right in the belly with her head.

It hurt. Christ, it hurt a lot. I wondered if I'd jolted the baby. But pregnant women routinely carry kicking, tantruming toddlers; get jostled on subways; even fall down stairs. Women are tough. The pain ebbed. I decided not to mention it to Tom.

Between races I nestled in a camp chair reading and snacking on fruit salad. I wasn't wearing maternity clothes yet, but my track pants were getting snug in their elastic waist. My belly was hard like a melon. Had it been like that before? I wondered if the baby could hear the dogs barking, and what she would make of such a noise. Would our infant daughter be conditioned to find the sound soothing, like a lullaby? As the afternoon wore on, finding a comfortable position grew more difficult. I shifted in the chair, keeping one eye on the race results and another on my iPhone Facebook feed, when I came to the realization that I was bleeding.

I willed myself not to overreact.

I dialed the doctor. The nurse who took the call was calm. Go get checked out, she said.

Is this an emergency? I asked.

Not necessarily, she said.

Tom

On the phone Kelley sounded strangely calm. She wasn't even sure I needed to rush over to get her. Muppet had another race coming up, and she thought maybe one of the other flyball teammates could give them a ride home. I didn't understand her lack of urgency. Hadn't we been trying to have this baby for years?

The St. Pete dog club was less than ten minutes away. When I arrived, Kelley said she wasn't in any pain and was not in any hurry. She insisted that we wait for Muppet's final run of the afternoon. Even though her teammates offered to take care of Muppet, she insisted that we drop our dog back at home ourselves.

"We need to get to the hospital as soon as possible," I said. "We need to find out what's wrong."

"Stop worrying," she said. "I'm only bleeding a little. I'll be fine."

By the time we dropped off Muppet, Kelley was grimacing. As we pulled out of our neighborhood, her face was clenched. She was fighting to catch her breath through the pain.

"Hurry," she told me.

I was doing everything but running red lights, but in minutes she had gone from mild discomfort to spasms sharp enough to make her cry out.

At the hospital, the nurses put her into a wheelchair right away and whisked her back to a triage room. Kelley's spasms were intensifying.

The obstetrician looked stricken when he entered the room. As Kelley clenched and vomited, he explained that if they couldn't stop the labor, our daughter had no chance of surviving outside the womb. But there was an even more pressing problem. Speaking quietly, the doctor explained to me that if amniotic fluid seeped into Kelley's bloodstream, the fluid might trigger a reaction that would make it harder to stop the hemorrhaging. They were giving her meds, but the meds weren't working.

"If we can't slow down the bleeding," he said, lowering his voice even further, "we might lose your wife."

Kelley grabbed my arm. Despite the doctor's best efforts, she had heard what he said.

"Don't let me die," she told me, tightening her grip as she stared into my face. "Please don't let me die."

For a moment I was speechless. I had never known Kelley to be afraid of anything. Now she was terrified, and I tried not to let her see how much it rattled me. Her cries were growing louder. Her face was turning white. The room was drenched in so much blood, it looked like a crime scene. Her pillow was dotted with vomited blueberries.

"I won't let you die," I whispered. "I promise. I'm right here."

Soon the drugs kicked in, and the hemorrhaging slowed. Now that Kelley was stabilized, the medical team checked on the baby. As they rolled in the ultrasound equipment, I tried to make my face as neutral as possible. I was sure our daughter was dead but did not want to suggest such a thing out loud.

A tech quickly ran a wand over Kelley's stomach, trying to

call up a heartbeat on the monitor. Nothing. The tech tried again, this time searching more thoroughly. I held my breath as she started on the right side, slowly moving the wand across every inch. Nothing. She moved to the center, below Kelley's navel. Nothing.

Kelley

I don't remember if I held my breath or gasped or spoke or sobbed. I remember the blood. Blood on my hands, blood on the bed. Blood in red rivulets and blood in dark clumps. Bright beads of blood on the doctor's blue latex gloves. Blood made redder by the fluorescence in the room. Blood made more horrible by my guilt. Blood in such startling quantity I knew absolutely that there was no baby, not anymore. Did Tom know yet? Did he know I had killed his daughter?

"I'm sorry," I told him. I writhed on the hospital bed, gripping the side rail, burying my face in its plastic indifference. "I'm so sorry."

He held my hand. There was blood on his hands. I had killed his baby, and the baby was dead, and now there was only this blood, from somewhere inside me where a baby should be, running out onto the floor.

I was toxic. Entrusted with the most precious thing in the world, the result of years of work and sacrifice by the people I most loved, I had fucked it all up. I had lost our baby. I looked at Tom. I could not lose him, too.

Here he was, a man who used to faint at the sight of a needle, spattered with my blood, upright, keeping his shit together. The gone baby had come from us. We still mattered. I promised myself we would be okay.

And then came the frozen shock when a heartbeat flooded the room, a sound like a galloping horse.

I must have felt relief, hearing that heartbeat. We still had a daughter, somehow. On the monitor, she bobbed and floated in the pixelated haze. But with that relief came a tide of fear. It felt crueler, somehow, to see her so content, so unaware, and know that one way or another, we were bound to watch her die.

In just a few hours, she had been lost and then found. Her heart pumped. She curled and wiggled. How quiet it must have been in there, in that warm pool. How safe she must have felt. But next to her loomed a mysterious shape that had not been there two days before: a clot of blood the size of a fist, created as the placenta had begun to tear loose from my body. A nurse pumped drugs into an IV to stall the labor, and gradually they took a tenuous hold. But it was clear to everyone that the reprieve was temporary. My baby and I were coming apart.

She couldn't live. Could she? I didn't want to ask. A normal pregnancy lasts forty weeks. I was only halfway there. If the doctors had not intervened, our baby would have been a second-trimester miscarriage.

Still caked in vomit and blood, I was wheeled to a private room. Over the next few days, I learned that early arrival kills more newborns than anything else, and complications from prematurity kill more babies in the first year than anything else. The doctors couldn't say when I would deliver. But if the baby came soon, the odds were awful.

For the next two or three weeks, she would be beyond rescue. If she were born, almost no doctor would intervene, because there was nothing he or she could do. Would our baby be just strong enough to struggle? Would she gasp? Breathe? Cry?

If I could stay pregnant for another five or six weeks, past twenty-five weeks gestation, almost all doctors would feel morally and legally obligated to try to save her life, studies showed. If I made it two months, to twenty-eight weeks, she would probably just spend a few weeks in the hospital learning to breathe and eat and then go home. I knew I wasn't making it to twenty-eight weeks.

In their calmest and firmest bedside voices, the doctors said I had to make it another month, to twenty-four weeks, loosely considered the earliest point of human viability outside the womb. At twenty-four weeks, a baby has a shot at survival. But it wasn't a great shot. And "survival" didn't guarantee quality of life. The scariest scenario was if I delivered right at that threshold—in the twenty-third week. Because that is the zone between viability and futility. New technologies might keep our daughter alive, but at great cost. Whether to try to save these infants was one of the fundamental controversies in medicine.

Bayfront Medical Center, the hospital where I lay monitored, was my home for the time being. But I didn't belong. The Labor and Delivery unit had been designed for celebrations. The rooms were private, with sleeping couches and flat-screen TVs. The hallways were lined with abstract roses, an extension of the fertility-clinic motif. Sliding panels obscured all evidence of the mess and peril of birth. Mothers were wheeled out holding fat, drowsy newborns, dutiful dads following with balloons. Every time a baby was born, the loudspeaker carried the tinkling of a lullaby.

It was easy to pretend, in this cozy place, that all babies came wailing into the world pink and robust, and were bundled and hatted and handed to teary mothers and proud dads. But behind the sliding panels in my room and in the delivery suites were hidden devices for oxygen, suction, and epinephrine. There was a morgue on the ground floor. And the Labor and Delivery unit, while officially part of Bayfront, was actually housed across the street inside an entirely different facility—All Children's Hospital. If a baby was born in trouble, as mine was bound to be, it was already in the place that cared for some of the sickest and most fragile children in the state.

When they sent me home, I lay still in bed and watched the calendar as my baby survived to twenty-one weeks, then twenty-two. Jennifer brought soft clothes and trashy magazines. I was not allowed to get out of bed even to go to the kitchen. Tom had a friend come to the house to cut my hair. I Googled pictures of half-formed babies. Most of the images were gruesome anti-abortion propaganda or shallow, superficial stories of "miracle babies" with tubes in their tracheas. They were both offensive. I did not need politics or false hope.

I saw at least a half-dozen doctors. My primary ob-gyn, Dr. Thomas McNeill, transferred me to a high-risk group, which put me at the mercy of a rotation of residents. Each one probed my nether regions and asked if I'd suffered any trauma. The questions became routine. Had I been hit by a car? Punched in the gut? Tom was usually in the room with me as I told them about the bike and the neighbor's idiot tumbleweed of a dog, and the doctors halfheartedly scribbled in their notes that a bike accident was the likely cause of the preterm labor. I did not mention the blunt instrument of Muppet's cranium ramming my belly at the flyball tournament. I still had not told Tom. I was afraid he would blame the dog or, worse, me. Maybe he would even leave me, when this was all over and we went home with no baby. Maybe he would decide that I was just too reckless to ever be anyone's mom.

The clot was not shrinking. On ultrasound it reminded me of a second baby, a blood baby, an evil twin. *Leave my daughter the fuck alone.*

"How bad is it?" I asked Dr. McNeill as he stopped in one day to check on me, even though I wasn't his patient anymore. He was direct.

"It's bad," he said. "You have a clot in your uterus the size of an orange. I'm very worried that you could lose this pregnancy."

Lose the pregnancy. Pregnancy is a condition. A noun. Synonym: gestation.

The baby was not the pregnancy. The baby was my daughter. *Lose my daughter.* She would slide out, wet, raw, mute, purple. Slide right out of my body in a river of my blood. She would not be lost at all, she would be right there, in my hands, turning gray.

I was fed a steady diet of pills to quiet my uterus. Still it quivered and bled. I began to see that sometimes doctors just don't know what to do. They were waiting for me to cross the twenty-four-week mark, and until I did, I was having a miscarriage.

On my second stay in the hospital, one tactless cherub of a doctor made the situation plain when he tried to discharge me. "Your baby is not viable," he said, "so you might as well deliver at home."

I had never seen this guy before, but he was ordering up

discharge papers. He wanted me to go home and bleed out on my own floor, and not tie up the hospital staff, who had more important, third-trimester patients to attend to. He must have seen the rage spread across my face.

"What's the matter?" he said. "Don't you understand the plan?"

Poor man. He was probably not even thirty. Just a resident whose mother had paid for MCAT prep but neglected to teach him social skills.

"I understand your plan," I said, summoning my iciest snarl. "Your plan sucks. Get out of my room, and don't come back until you have a better fucking plan."

I was shaking when he left. People in lab coats were supposed to have answers. Whatever was wrong with me was not in their textbooks.

I bloated and swelled from being stuck in bed so long. I had to wear strange hospital compression socks and pee in a bedpan. Tom and I discovered it was impossible to stay miserable around the clock. We watched Netflix and amused ourselves by speculating about the romantic lives of the doctors and nurses. One doctor looked like a lost Kennedy. Another kept the nurses laughing; we could hear them out in the hall. Our favorite was a chestnut-haired nurse we called Cupcake who wore *Grey's Anatomy*–label scrubs. I imagined all of them screwing in supply closets and gossiping at the nurses' station. One handsome doctor, while sketching a diagram of the untenable situation in my uterus, asked if I had any questions.

"Just one," I said. "Is it me or are the people on this floor unusually hot?"

"Yes," he said, "and thank God for it."

All of these people had been between my legs, and I was too

wrecked to care. The absurdity of it made me laugh, even though laughter was discouraged while on bed rest.

By the twenty-third week, I was taunted by the incessant lullaby on the hospital loudspeaker, a reminder of how natural this process was supposed to be. I stayed anchored to the hospital bed by a strap around my belly that charted the volcanic activity within on a computer monitor. The contractions came and went, and when they got bad enough, the doctors stalled the labor by elevating my feet above my head and flooding me with magnesium sulfate, which made me feel like my blood and skin were on fire. That's how I was—inverted, scalding—when doctors conceded the baby was coming soon, and a neonatologist visited to advise Tom and me of what lay ahead.

Dr. Aaron Germain was thin and kind, with a look of constant worry. I viewed him as an ambassador from the Land of Sick Babies, a place I could not imagine.

He knew how badly we wanted our child, he told us, and an army of specialists with the most advanced technology was ready upstairs to try to save her life. But we needed to decide whether saving her was what we really wanted. The effort would require months of aggressive intervention and could leave us with a child who was alive, but very damaged.

Few doctors would insist on intervening. The choice was ours to make.

He went through the list of possible calamities, each with its own initials. IVH, PFO, RDS, CLD, ROP, CP. The magnesium sulfate burned through me. *Blood in the brain. Hole in the heart. Respiratory distress. Chronic lung disease. Ventilator. Wheelchair. Blind. Deaf. Developmental delays. Autism. Seizures. Cerebral palsy.*

Every part of her was underdeveloped and weak. Every

treatment would exact a toll. She might live, but she would likely have, to use the medical term, profound morbidities.

Odds she would die, no matter how hard they tried: better than half.

Odds she would die or be seriously disabled: 68 percent.

Odds she would die or be at least moderately disabled: 80 percent.

There was a 20 percent chance she would live and be reasonably okay. I pictured her in the slow class at school, battling asthma or peering through thick glasses. We would buy her pink sparkly ones and tell her they were cool.

I contemplated that figure: 20 percent. It didn't seem hopeless. Then again, imagine a revolver with five chambers. Now put four bullets in it and play Russian roulette. Would we bet on a 20 percent chance if losing might mean forfeiting everything we cared about? Would we torture our baby with aggressive treatment just so she could live out her life in a nursing home or on a ventilator? Would we lose our house? Would our marriage fall apart?

Dr. Germain gamely counseled us as we searched for loopholes in the statistics. Girls did better than boys, he said, but white babies like ours fared worse than black babies. Before the birth, I would be injected with steroids to strengthen our daughter's lungs. She would be delivered by C-section so her body wouldn't get mangled in the birth canal.

But what were the odds, we wanted to know, for a middle-class girl baby with good parents who sing songs and read stories? A girl with two big brothers and aunts and uncles and a friendly, big-eared dog? The baby who slumbered inside me, her heartbeat hammering along over the speakers, reminding us that she was perfectly fine in there, and safe, and how wrong it was that soon she would be wrenched into the bright, cold air and made to breathe?

Dr. Germain spoke softly and didn't rush. He was a smart man, and doing his best. I wanted him to tell us what to do.

He couldn't say. The answers we wanted were not in the data.

"The statistics don't matter," he said, "until they happen to you."

What echoed in my head was something Dr. Germain never said: saving her might be the most selfish act in the world.

Tom

The doctor explained the probabilities with great patience, the words tripping gently from his mouth. Was he relying on a protocol he'd seen on a PowerPoint?

From where I stood next to the window, I could see the palm trees three floors below, swaying beside the hospital parking lot, and the cars easing down the street, their drivers going about their lives, and the sun setting over the Gulf, and the day aglow, and yet through it all, I was seized by Dr. Germain's maddening calm. He was telling us to let our daughter die. He hadn't said those words, but it's what I heard. He thought we should kill our baby.

Kelley, still lying in the bed, was asking all the questions. I could barely say anything, because I was trying so hard to compose myself. I was not a violent person. I'd been in only one fist-fight in my life, back in seventh grade, when a kid hit me with a whip. But now my jaw was tightening and my hands were clenching. I wanted to knock this man to the ground and beat the logic out of him forever.

He reminded me of Eeyore. His sad eyes, his woebegone posture. The way he spoke with practiced resignation. In my head, I heard myself calling him Dr. Eeyore, and the idea was so stupid that it interrupted the loop of my vengeful thoughts.

We needed to decide, quickly, whether to ask them to resuscitate her when she was born. Preferably that night. Because no matter what the doctors tried, the baby was coming. She would be born sometime in the next forty-eight hours, he said, and he thought it best if we were ready.

"Once you see her," he said, "it will be too hard."

Kelley

After the doctor left, Tom sat on the edge of the bed and held my hand. I could feel our baby kicking and turning. I would do anything to save her. I would stop time. I would give my life. I would give my arm to buy her another month. But the doctor's litany of disability was chilling. What if she didn't want to be saved?

I had to scoff at my expectations. We were a family of high achievers. Tom was a Pulitzer Prize–winning writer. Nat and Sam were salutatorian and valedictorian, respectively, at Gibbs High. Now they were off at college. We had envisioned a similar path for our daughter—horseback riding, guitar lessons, and the dean's list. All that was gone now, and we grappled with the fundamentals. If she lived, would she walk or talk? Would she one day give us a look that said, *Why did you put me through this?*

People always ask me if I prayed. I prayed the way people in foxholes are said to pray. I prayed with every thought and every breath. And I prayed with the certainty that I had no business praying, that I hadn't earned the right. I'd never been religious. Worse, I knew we had defied the natural order in our determination to have a child. Through so many in vitro procedures, with so many tests and needles and vials of drugs, we'd created life in a dish. To be given a child just long enough to watch her die felt like punishment for our hubris.

I was crying when I asked Tom, "Did we want her too much?"

I don't remember sleeping that night. As dawn crept closer, we both swallowed the thing we couldn't say. I knew once I said it our baby would be gone, and we'd be the parents who had turned our backs. Tom climbed in next to me on the skinny bed and wrapped his arms around me and all of the wires as best he could.

"I don't know how to do this," he said.

Our baby's heart kept beating. I held out my iPhone and used its recorder to capture the sound, in case it was the only evidence of my daughter I would ever have.

I'm here, it kept telling us. *I'm still here.*

The next day, a second emissary arrived from the neonatal intensive care unit. Nurse Practitioner Diane Loisel found us still choking on indecision and grief.

Diane had a relaxed, no-makeup look, a contrast to the crisp, professional bearing of the neonatologist. *Given the stakes,* I thought, *could we get the doctor back in here?* As soon as Diane started to talk, I felt foolish. She was so straightforward, it was clear her only priority was our baby.

Diane told us she had worked with small and sick babies for thirty years. When she started, twenty-three-weekers never made it out of the delivery room. Any baby born weighing less than 1,000 grams—about 2 pounds—was considered not viable and allowed to die. But now science had advanced, raising new questions for everybody.

Some parents insisted the doctors do everything possible,

then insisted on the impossible, too. Diane told us it sometimes made her angry to see tiny babies subjected to futile intervention, to see them go into nursing homes or to families ill equipped to care for them. The more educated parents asked more questions, considered quality of life. Diane often wondered if pushing parents to make such life-and-death decisions was cruel.

When it came to babies born at twenty-three weeks, research showed, there was little consensus from one hospital to the next or even among doctors working the same shift in the same unit.

Some of these micro-preemies were born limp and blue, and some came out pink and crying. In those first hours and days, much could be revealed. And there was a window of time, while the baby was on a ventilator and still very fragile, when doctors and families could reverse course and withdraw life support.

"You don't have to decide right now," Diane said. "It's a process."

She seemed to be offering an escape from the torment we had suffered all night, an end to the unbearable coin toss. We could let them intervene and see how it went. If our baby was born too weak, we could decide later to let her go.

"We don't want her to suffer," Tom said. "But we want our baby to have a chance."

As Diane headed back to the NICU, she told me later, she knew she had changed everything. She also knew that once a mother had seen her baby for the first time, there often was no turning back. She hoped we wouldn't blame her for the rest of our lives.

That afternoon we watched TV and allowed ourselves to hope the doctors were wrong and we would make it another week. As soon as the sky darkened outside the window, I tried to sleep, to make the day end before anything could ruin it.

Still tethered like Gulliver by IVs and wires, I shifted left, then back to the right. Adjusted the bed up and back down. Stole Tom's pillow and asked the nurse for extra blankets. A vague unease settled in, and I shut my eyes and willed it away. The monitor registered no unusual activity.

When the nurse came in for yet another blood-pressure reading, I told her I felt strange.

Constipation, she said.

At first it was uncomfortable. Then it started to hurt.

Tom

The spasms started at midnight. They rolled through Kelley's body and stopped and then started again. But the monitor showed no sign of contractions, and no matter what we said, the nurse would not budge. Kelley had an order for morphine "as needed," but the nurse refused to give her so much as an aspirin.

As the waves intensified, I grew frantic. I told the nurse that Kelley had an unusually high pain tolerance and I had never seen her suffer like this. How on earth could this be constipation?

"Oh, I've seen it before," the nurse said. The only thing that would help my wife, she insisted, was prune juice.

"You're serious," I said.

"Yes. You need to get some for her as quickly as possible."

The hospital cafeteria downstairs was closed, she added.

"What about the morphine?" I said.

"No, she needs prune juice."

Out I went, running toward our car. By now it was 2:00 a.m. St. Petersburg was a quiet town. Most groceries closed at 9:00 p.m. Then I remembered the Sweetbay on MLK Street North, only a few minutes away. Though I'd never shopped there this late, I remembered the sign in front saying they were open twenty-four hours. I sped as fast as I could, rehearsing what I would say if the cops pulled me over. Would they assume I was drunk? Was it possible that they had encountered other dads on other nights, tearing through the city on a quest for prune juice?

When I pulled up in front of Sweetbay, the doors were locked. I could see a man inside, his back to me, polishing the floors as he listened to headphones. But the rest of the store appeared empty. When had they changed their hours?

I hit the gas again and cut across Thirty-eighth Avenue toward the Albertsons on Fourth Street. For as long as I'd lived in St. Pete, they had been open all night. But now Albertsons was closed, too. What the hell was going on? Had every grocery in the city cut back its hours? I was yelling and cursing and pounding my steering wheel like Popeye Doyle in *The French Connection*. But Doyle had been chasing a murderer. All I wanted was for my wife to stop hurting.

By now even the bars were closing. The streets were deserted, almost desolate. The houses I passed looked haunted. The solitude reminded me of the midnight drives I had made to Kelley's house, so long before. The feeling that I was in a dream where the rest of the world had vanished. The sense that I was becoming a ghost without substance or consequence. But tonight I was overwhelmed not by guilt but by a sense of impotence. I couldn't stand Kelley being in such pain. From the odds we had been quoted, I knew that our unborn child probably would not live through another day. And yet I was away from them both, careening through the city on this absurd mission.

The next stop was a 7-Eleven. It was open, but when I hurried inside, the clerk told me they didn't carry prune juice. Back in the car, more yelling and cursing. This time I cut west for a CVS at the corner of Twenty-second Avenue and U.S. 19. I couldn't think of anyplace else. If they weren't open, I had no idea where to go next.

As I screeched into the parking lot, I saw the lighted sign and customers walking in and out of the front doors.

"Thank God."

I tore inside. The clerk directed me to the food aisle, where prune juice awaited. I grabbed a sixty-four-ounce bottle, the biggest they had, along with a box of prunes for good measure. I could not remember the last time I'd showered. My eyes were bloodshot; my wild silver hair resembled a fright wig. When the clerk took my credit card, she stared at me as though I was a lunatic.

Kelley

The pain was sharp and low, and I could feel the baby kicking with both feet, like a mule trying to take down a barn door. "Please," I told her. "Be still."

I was crouched on the bathroom floor. It was cold and smelled of hospital soap. The toilet-paper holder at eye level spit out individual sheets, like Kleenex, and I thought, *How stupid that I'm going to remember that detail for the rest of my life.*

On the toilet was a plastic container to catch the blood that was leaking out of me. It came out in clots, and each one felt like a baby part. I was afraid to look anymore. I didn't want my daughter to be born in pieces into a hospital toilet, so I moved to the floor.

I shifted from my back to my knees to a crouch and back again. My daughter was not listening to me. Perhaps that is what daughters did. They learned the hard way. She would fall out onto this dirty tile, slippery and angry, and what would I do? We were so alone. Tom was on some ludicrous expedition. The nurse was doing whatever nurses do when they are not calling the goddamn doctor.

"Baby, baby, please be still." I was whispering, out loud. I clutched the IV pole. I clenched my teeth and screamed.

"Please, baby, stay safe. Go to sleep."

The nurse appeared in the doorway. "What would it feel like if there were feet coming out of me?" I asked her. "Because that's what this feels like."

"No, honey," she assured me. "That's not what's happening." She was gone again.

Tom

I heard the screams even before I opened the door.

Kelley was asking me why I had been gone so long and why the pain wouldn't stop. I wanted to tell her everything was going to be fine, but she would have known I was lying. Instead I hit the call button and wiped her face with a wet cloth, brushed her hair out of her eyes, poured some prune juice into a cup, and helped her sip. We hadn't yet taken the Lamaze classes, but I remembered the lessons from when Nat was born, so I tried to get her to breathe with me. She was too panicked.

"This isn't right," she kept saying. "Something is wrong. Something is wrong. I know something is wrong."

The next wave was coming. Her grip tightened on my hand. Soon her eyes were closing, and her mouth was widening into an O, and her face was growing more and more rigid until it shattered with her cries. She had my hand in a death grip now and was pulling like she wanted to wrench it off. Finally the nurse appeared in the doorway. She seemed impatient, irritated. Why hadn't I given my wife the prune juice?

We pointed toward the open bottle and asked her to check the monitor again. The nurse sighed and did it. Still no signs of contractions.

"Are you sure?" Kelley said. "Is it working?"

The nurse said the equipment was fine. Kelley asked again for the morphine. She asked if someone could page a doctor. No need for either, said the nurse. Once the prune juice kicked in, everything would be fine.

She disappeared, and another wave took hold. During a lull between the spasms, I ran out to the nurse's station and told her something was terribly wrong, no matter what the monitor showed or didn't show, and insisted she get a doctor right away. She sighed again.

Eventually a young resident showed up. When he saw how much Kelley was suffering, he snapped a glove onto his hand to check her cervix. She was sobbing now and gulping for air, and she asked him to not do anything that would hurt the baby. He told her to be still and breathe.

"Please be careful," Kelley said. "Please be careful, please be careful."

The room was dark, but when the resident stood up, enough light poured in from the hall that I could see the startled look on his face. The nurse saw it, too. By now it was almost dawn. Kelley had been screaming off and on for more than two hours.

Another resident materialized, someone more senior, and when she checked Kelley, a look came over her face, too.

"We have to get you to an operating room," she said.

Kelley was breathing so hard she seemed on the verge of passing out. Twenty-four weeks. They had told us the baby had no chance unless we made it to twenty-four weeks. We were now at twenty-three weeks and six days. She begged the doctor to do something, anything, to delay the delivery.

Put me in a coma, she said. Wake me up when the baby is bigger.

The doctor shook her head.

"The bag is coming out," she said. "I could feel two feet kicking."

Just as Kelley had described.

"Couldn't you just sew me shut? Maybe hang me upside down? Just don't let my baby be born yet."

It destroyed me, seeing her scrabble for more time. Better than anyone, I knew the ferocity of this woman's will to be a mother. But I had never seen it expressed so nakedly, with such desperation.

Speaking softly, the doctor explained that our daughter was so premature and fragile that an emergency C-section was the only option. She was coming out breech. If the rest of her body was squeezed through the birth canal, the doctor said, the blood vessels in her head might rupture.

"I'm sorry, sweetie. We have to go now."

They put Kelley on a gurney and let me walk alongside as they took her downstairs to surgery. She looked so pale and terrified. I could see Dr. Germain's statistics ticking in her head, as they were ticking in mine.

"My baby," she kept saying. "Please help my baby."

At the double doors leading to the O.R., they told me to wait. The team needed to prep her and give her a spinal, and then they would come get me. I paced back and forth and thought about Nat and Sam, still asleep and unaware that their little sister was crashing her way into the world. I wondered if she would live long enough for them to meet her, if she would have the chance to look in their faces and hear their voices. The thought made me gasp.

A nurse came out and handed me scrubs to pull over my clothes and shoes. She told me I would be with my wife shortly.

I had only the vaguest notion of the time. I looked at my phone.

Juniper

Tuesday, April 12.
5:59 a.m.

The doors opened, and the nurse motioned me back. I saw Kelley stretched out on the table, the doctors gathered around her in their blue masks, the bright light beaming a circle of pure white onto her belly. A roaring filled my ears. A rushing sound, like a mad wind. This is what it must be like, I told myself, to jump out of a plane.

Kelley

I heard voices. The doctors were talking about a movie they had seen. I wanted to yell at them to focus, because didn't they realize that a half-formed human was being ripped from my body, and that she might only have right now, these few minutes or hours, and wasn't that enough to get their attention? But I couldn't yell. I held Tom's hand. I turned my head toward him and threw up.

I could see the giant round light above us, a hovering spaceship. In the hall, I'd heard the doctors wondering aloud whether there was time for anesthesia. Then they'd hastily rolled me on my side and stuck a needle in my spine, and the numbness had washed over me like warm water.

If I'd been able to sit up and look around, I would have seen a group from the NICU, called the Stork Team, preparing to stabilize the baby in a room next to the O.R.

Gwen Newton was the Stork Team nurse that day. She described it all for me later. She said most mornings, she needed a good jolt of coffee to get going. But that day, all it took was a look at her assignment sheet: *twenty-three-weeker.* When she was pregnant with her son, she'd had nightmares that he'd been born at twenty-three weeks.

She readied a mobile incubator that would keep the baby

warm and monitored on the short ride to the NICU. She made a nest of blankets and spread a pillowcase over it to catch the blood.

The baby's arm would be so small she'd use a rubber band for a tourniquet. She got out a No. 1 blood-pressure cuff, small enough to fit around her own finger. She set the warmer to 37 degrees Celsius, laid out catheters for IVs and wires for monitors. She drew a mixture of 5 percent dextrose in a 60-milliliter syringe—a snack to get the baby started. And she drew 1.4 milliliters of an artificial lung surfactant, a mix of fats and proteins to help prevent the baby's sticky lungs from collapsing.

A respiratory therapist was prepping the ventilator, and a neonatologist and a nurse practitioner were studying the chart. When Gwen had everything ready, she stepped to the doorway to watch the C-section.

Some of what happened next would be out of her control. Some babies came out fighting and some did not. *You never know what's coming out of that belly,* she thought.

I felt a sickening tug. I knew that we were two separate people now.

"She's kicking," Tom said. He was peering over the surgical drape at the gaping red meat of my abdomen, and at the unfinished child that had just emerged from it. Someone said she cried, but I didn't hear it. I tasted prune vomit in my mouth.

Gwen took the tiny blood-spotted bundle from the delivery nurse. She unwrapped her, laid her on heat packs, and slipped her into a plastic bag up to her neck to help prevent heat and fluid loss. Gwen rubbed and dried her like a mother cat roughs up a kitten, but more gently, so as not to tear her skin. The baby was dusky blue, then dark red. Gwen pinched the tiny greenish umbilical cord between her thumb and forefinger and felt it throb. She counted seventeen beats in six seconds.

"Heart rate is one seventy," she called out. It was strong, a good sign.

The baby was trying to breathe, but her lungs were not ready and her muscles were weak. Through the stethoscope her breathing sounded squeaky and coarse. A respiratory therapist threaded a tube the size of thick spaghetti through her mouth and into her chest. Into the tube she placed the milky fluid that would coat the baby's lungs. She connected her to a small portable ventilator that delivered oxygen at a constant pressure and tapped her finger over a hole in the tube to pace the breaths. The baby's chest heaved mechanically.

She weighed 570 grams—1 pound 4 ounces. She was 11.4 inches long—the length of a Barbie doll.

I was still staring at the spaceship light overhead when someone slipped a piece of paper in front of me, and an ink pad, and asked for a fingerprint. On the paper were two still-wet footprints, each an inch and a half long. Startling evidence that she was here.

"My baby," I kept saying, "my baby, my baby."

I saw Gwen roll the incubator past. Inside was a raw dark blur in a too-big hat. Tom looked at me and looked at the baby.

"Go with her," I said. "Please go."

Tom

I rode the elevator, wrapped inside myself, trembling. If anyone else rode with me, I didn't notice. The recorded voices of children announced when it was time to get on and off, but I didn't hear them. I was thinking about Nat's and Sam's births, the tsunami that had swept through me when I first saw them. But my sons had both been seven-pounders, fat and squawking.

In the delivery room, I had glimpsed my daughter's beet-red skin glowing in the surgical light, sticklike arms and legs, the scrunched and angry face of a homunculus. An unkind thought, but it was what came to mind. Beyond that, I wasn't sure what she looked like. I had seen photos of micro-preemies this size, and the images had frightened me. What if I couldn't bond with her? What if I didn't recognize her as my daughter?

"Sixth floor," announced one of the children's voices.

The elevator opened. A sign directed me to the right, toward a set of locked doors. I pressed a button on an intercom and the receptionist buzzed me in. It felt as though I were entering a biohazard lab.

"The pod is this way," she said, leading me around a corner and down another hallway and then pressing her badge against a sensor to allow us through a second set of security doors.

She left me standing at the threshold of a large room that seemed stolen from science fiction. A dozen incubators lined the walls, each plastic box holding a tiny creature, each creature connected by multiple wires to looming banks of machines. Alarms were pinging and beeping; red and yellow lights were flashing. Some of the incubators were closed, with quilts draped over the tops. Inside I could make out the shadowy outlines of the patients, curled and sleeping. Other incubators were open, their oblong lids raised several feet into the air, and teams of people in scrubs huddled over the squirming occupants.

A nurse told me I had to sanitize my hands before I could enter. Micro-preemies had almost no immune systems, she said. Germs could kill them. At the wash station, I took off my wedding ring and pumped soap into my hands. Across the room, I could see the nurse and neonatologist who had brought our daughter up here leaning over one of the open boxes.

As I walked toward them, the room spun and swayed. Everything was slowing down and speeding up. I made my feet walk to the edge of the box and made my eyes look inside. She was lying naked on a plastic sheet layered over the pillowcase and the blankets, her head cradled in some kind of curved pillow and her arms reaching in either direction, fingers splayed. The plastic, smeared with blood, crinkled as the nurse from the delivery room lifted her to wrap a measuring tape around her stomach.

"Can you write sixteen for the girth now, please?" Gwen was saying to someone.

"The girth?"

"Yeah."

I could not stop shaking. When the nurses reached in to touch her, their hands looked giant. Her skin was papyrus, and beneath I could see the web of her veins, spidering up her arms and into her hands and her long anemone fingers. Everything about her declared that she still belonged inside her mother.

Alarms kept sounding, and nurses and techs were weaving back and forth in a choreography of controlled urgency.

"She looks much better than she did initially," the neonatologist said.

"Yup," said Gwen.

When there was a spare moment, the neonatologist introduced herself. Dr. Jeane McCarthy was maybe seventy, so wizened that she reminded me of Yoda. This was comforting, because Yoda knows what he's doing.

The doctor told me that the team was doing everything they could. She didn't tell me, until much later, that after working with thousands of babies over four decades, she was not sure this one would make it. If it had been her baby, she would not have resuscitated.

For the moment, she kept these opinions to herself and stepped away.

Gwen finished taping one of the baby's lines and closed the top of the incubator. She offered me hand sanitizer and sat me down on a stool beside the box and told me I could touch my daughter, if I wanted.

"Will it hurt her?"

"Not if you're careful."

Gwen showed me how. She told me not to rub back and forth, or else the skin might slough off. She opened a porthole on the side of the box so I could reach inside. Then she left me there alone with the baby.

I took a deep breath, then slowly reached in with my left hand and placed the tip of my little finger in her right palm. At once she grabbed on. The power of her grip humbled me. Why was I so afraid, when she was so strong? I sat there, my shoulders heaving. I thought about everything she had been through in the past twelve hours. Surely she had heard her mother's screams with the contractions and had felt the hand of the doctor against her kicking feet. Had it hurt when they pulled her into the light? What could she possibly make of what was happening now?

I was swept away. I saw her will, her beauty, all the possibilities waiting inside her. She was a work in progress, yes. So was I.

"Hey, Peanut," I whispered. "It's Daddy."

Kelley

A baby at twenty-three weeks gestation has begun to hear but can't yet see. It may detect its mother's voice. It has a dawning awareness of whether it is right side up or upside down. The surface of its brain is smooth, just beginning to develop the hills and valleys that become wrinkles and folds. The baby responds to pain but has no capacity for memory or for complex thought. Its lungs look like scrawny saplings compared to the full, bushy trees of normal lungs. Its bones are soft. It swallows. Its hair and eyelashes are starting to grow, and its fingernails and fingerprints are forming. Its body is covered with a soft protective down. It is recognizably human, but barely.

I was still in recovery when Tom returned from the NICU.

"She's perfect," he said. His voice was a squeak. "She's so beautiful."

I just stared at him. My sweet, emotional husband, in the grip of something elemental and overwhelming. He'd been to a place I couldn't fathom.

"That's my baby girl up there," he kept saying. "That's my daughter."

He showed me a cell phone photo, but it didn't register. I

was sedated, I guess, or in shock. I knew I would see her soon, and I was afraid. I watched the clock.

Tom said she was perfect. He had to be out of his mind.

I used to imagine what I would say to her when I first saw her. She'd be wrapped in a blanket and wearing a hat, and she'd feel solid in my arms, like a puppy. She might open one eye and peek up at me, perplexed but curious. She would know my voice and my smell, know I was her mother, and because she knew those things, she would not be afraid. I'd be hit with a force that would unmake me and remake me, right there.

Instead I waited while she fought for her life somewhere beyond my reach. She must have needed me. I must have let her down. After a hazy seven hours, the nurses said I was stable enough, and Tom took me to the NICU in a wheelchair, still in my cotton surgical gown, lugging an IV pole.

Tom pushed my wheelchair up to the deep sink so I could wash my hands. There were posted instructions and a disposable scrub brush, and I felt determined to do it properly, for the full thirty seconds, in the hottest possible water, as if precise compliance with the rules might tip the odds.

I saw her plastic box halfway across the room. I didn't see anything else, just this tunnel of space and time and of everything changing that marked the distance between us. Here I was one person, and there I would become someone else. The soap was hard to rinse, and I let the water run for a long time.

Tom wheeled me forward. There, through the clear plastic, was my daughter. She was red and angular, angry like a fresh wound. She had a black eye and bruises on her body. Tubes snaked out of her mouth, her belly button, her hand. Wires moored her to monitors. Tape obscured her face. Her chin was long and narrow, her mouth agape because of the tubes. Dried blood crusted the corner of her mouth and the top of her diaper. The diaper was smaller than a playing card, and it swallowed her. She had no body fat, so she resembled a shrunken old man, missing his teeth. Her skin was nearly translucent, and through her chest I could see the beat of her flickering heart.

She kicked and jerked. She stretched her arms wide, palms open, as if in welcome or surrender.

I recognized her. I knew the shape of her head and the curve of her butt. I knew the strength of her kick. I knew how she had fit inside me and felt an acute sensation that she had been cut out, and of how wrong that was. I would do anything to put her back inside, to keep her safe.

"Hello, baby.

"It's Mommy."

Crazy questions flashed through my mind. Should we prepare a birth announcement? What would we name her? If she died, would we get a birth certificate? Would there be a funeral? Would we get a box of ashes, and if so, what size box? Was she aware of us? Did she recognize me like I recognized her? Was she afraid? Did she wonder where I had gone? If she ever got out of this box, would she know I was her mother?

She was alien and familiar. She was terrifying and beautiful. She was complete and interrupted. I felt the icy hush that comes with looking at a secret you are not meant to see. I was peeking into God's pocket.

"You can touch her," the nurse said.

I reached in through the porthole. I saw how white and swollen my hand was. I let it hover over her for a second, then pulled away, as if from a fire. Finally I placed the tip of my pinkie into her tiny palm.

She grabbed on.

PART THREE

Zero Zone

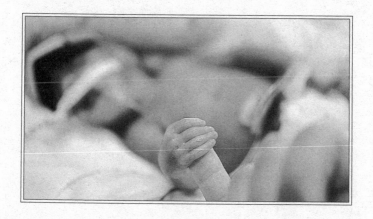

Kelley

Somewhere in this place my new daughter lay alone, struggling to breathe. I could feel the stabbing incision where they had cut her out of me two days before. That's how it felt—as if there had been an assault, perhaps in an alley with a dull spoon. The doctors had been kind and correct, and they'd had no choice. But they might as well have taken my liver, or my heart.

The curving pastel hallways felt infinite. I'd visited her—a raw and tiny thing—but could not remember how to get back there, and I wasn't supposed to go alone. It was night, and Tom had gone home to sleep. I would not be discharged for a few more days.

I clutched a syringe containing a trace amount of milk. Since her birth, I'd spent nearly every hour in a hospital bed attached to an electric breast pump, a frustrating and painful exercise that only magnified the absurdity of the situation. My body did not seem to know what to do. It was April 2011 and the baby wasn't due until August, yet here she was. Everything was out of sync.

I had wrung out a few drops and collected them in this syringe, the kind you'd use to feed an orphaned squirrel. It was a pathetic amount, but the nurses insisted the baby needed every drop. Her underdeveloped gut was vulnerable to infection and rupture. My milk could coat her stomach lining with protective antibodies. The pressure to produce the stuff was immense. If one more nurse called it liquid gold, I was going to spit.

The odds said she would die. I wondered how much time we had. I couldn't hold her or feed her. I didn't know if she was aware of me at all. I could do nothing to help her, or even to assert myself as her mother, except deliver this milk.

My insides screamed. Vicodin had been prescribed, but I had skipped the dose because I wanted to keep drugs out of the milk. I came to the long window of what I thought of as the Fat Baby Nursery. This was the place for healthy newborns—goliaths who wailed petty complaints with robust lungs. "What's your problem, Fatty?" I said to one. No nine-pounder had any right to complain.

I took a staff elevator up three floors. At a pair of locked double doors I picked up a phone. "I'm here to visit my daughter," I said.

Daughter.

The word was so unfamiliar it caught in my throat.

Inside, a nurse guided me to her and took the milk from my hand.

"Is it enough?" I asked.

It was one milliliter, a thimbleful, but just enough for a baby so small. The nurse attached it to the tube snaking into the baby's mouth and down to her belly.

It was gone in a second.

Over the next day or so, as the shock and sedatives wore off, I could see her better. She lay under a blue light, because of jaundice, which made her seem all the more surreal. She was so fragile that even delicate handling had left her battered. All her fine details—hair, eyelids, fingernails—looked slightly blurry, like a partially developed Polaroid. Her head was smaller than a tennis ball. Her ears had no cartilage, so they crumpled. She had no nipples—they wouldn't form for a few more weeks. The ventilator made her belly heave with such force her chest dimpled under the ribs. Wires sprouted from electrodes on her chest. A red sensor glowed on her foot. An IV ran into her hand. A wheeled pole next to her bed was stacked with three levels of pumps dosing out caffeine, antibiotics, pain medication, and sedatives. A hanging bag contained liquid intravenous nutrition, precisely calibrated each day. She was so obscured by tape and technology that I struggled to imagine her naked face. Her fingers and feet were mesmerizing. Impossibly long and exquisite, they shocked me every time they moved.

I texted a photo of her feet to Jennifer. Jennifer texted me back a photo of her own bare foot, her tanned toes flexing toward the camera.

I have perfect feet, she wrote. I had never noticed Jennifer's feet, but there they were, apparently, replicated in this new person.

This baby had been created with the genetic instructions for another woman's foot. She curled her fingers around her thumb, forming a fist. I always made a fist with the thumb outside, so if I ever had to punch someone, I would not break my thumb. I never had actually punched anyone, but this was my reasoning. Tom's sister had told me that her mother made a fist with her thumb on the inside. Was that genetics, too?

She had Jennifer's feet and eyebrows and nose. She had her grandmother's fist. She had lived inside my body, so she had my blood type. But then she'd been snatched away at birth, and the umbilical cord connecting us was cut and replaced with lines connecting her to machines.

Would I ever find my way back to her? Was I really a mother now? Was *mother* a noun or a verb, and what did it mean, in this strange place?

Before, there had been only my baby in my body. But looking around, now I was immersed in a multimillion-dollar artificial womb. The work of my balking uterus was replicated by an army of specialists in a facility that looked like an alien hive.

There were rows of incubators covered with quilts to shut out light and sound. I studied the one that held my baby. It was a GE Giraffe OmniBed, so most people called it the Giraffe. It had double Plexiglas walls and two portholes on each side. The lid raised and lowered on a mechanical arm, and the walls folded down for access. With radiant heat and circulating air, it kept the temperature and humidity constant even when the doors opened. The pressure-sensitive mattress tilted and spun like a lazy Susan. It could record her weight and temperature, allow for X-rays and even surgery.

Inside it, the baby reminded me of a chicken nugget under the heat lamp at McDonald's.

Hi, Nugget.

I couldn't see or approach the other babies, though I wanted to. I expected to hear crying, but babies didn't cry here. Their faces contorted in protest, but the tubes in their throats stopped the sound. The machines beeped and alarmed. The room swarmed with people in scrubs. Here and there sat bleary parents in various stages of boredom and shock. I did not know my place in this new world.

The NICU was a technological triumph. Science had made life possible at earlier and earlier stages of development, but inside those possibilities, terrible bargains were made. Medicine, ambition, compassion, and common sense collided here every day.

Another parent once called it the Zero Zone, and when I heard that, my mind flooded with context and understanding. It was a place that existed outside of time, apart from everything I used to know and from the person I used to be. It was as if I'd been jerked out of my own shoes, out of the life I recognized. Every second was an improbable gift and an agonizing eternity. Would my baby die today? Would she die before lunch? If I left for an hour, would she die while I was gone? There was no future, no past. There was only a desperate struggle to maintain.

The Zero Zone. The idea became hypnotic, took on multiple interpretations. Our baby was born at a unique window of time, at twenty-three weeks and six days gestation. She was an averted miscarriage, not yet fully her own person with her own standing. Because the questions were so unanswerable, the decision to put her on life support and allow her a chance to live had belonged to Tom and me, not the doctors and not the state.

This place was a frontier. Between life and death, certainly, but also between right and wrong, and between who we used to be and who we were becoming.

Our daughter occupied Bed 692, in the middle of the pod. On Wednesday, a nurse practitioner stopped by to lift the quilt and peer at the day-old baby inside. We were frozen and numb, but we recognized her as Diane, the person who'd led us to the decision not to let our baby go. I felt solid ground for the first time in days. Here was someone we could relate to. She talked to us like real people, not patients. She was warmth in a sterile place.

Our baby was a tiny thing, Diane said, but wiggly. That was

a decent sign. She opened a porthole and used a stethoscope the size of a quarter to listen to the baby's lungs. They sounded clear on both sides. She looked at the ventilator settings. The baby was receiving 21 percent oxygen—the same amount as in the air around us. Excellent.

Diane heeded her instinct as she moved from baby to baby, she said. Something about this baby encouraged her. The first week, though, was often called the honeymoon period. She warned us that things could turn in a flash.

We reminded her that we did not want to torture our baby with futile treatment.

Diane nodded. "She looks good for now."

"But you'll let us know when to freak out, right?" I said.

"I will tell you when to freak out."

There were ninety-seven beds like this one, taking up an entire floor of the hospital. The plumper preemies and the mildly sick—the "feeders and growers"—went to the north side. The more critical—the ones with ventilators or seizures or a hiccup in their chromosomes—came here to Six South. Most babies had private rooms, but a dozen shared this open space on the far west end of the building.

I asked, later, and learned that ninety babies were admitted that April. About a quarter were drug babies—oxycodone, methadone—and the rest were genetic disorders, birth defects, and preemies. Over time we became aware of babies with missing limbs, holes in their spines, shunts in their brains. Two babies were born that month at the edge of viability. I never saw the other one.

Parents were oddly scarce. The chairs by many of the incubators stayed empty. All Children's took babies from as far away as the Caribbean. Some parents couldn't make the trip. Some were in prison or rehab, and some, faced with the fragility and complexity of life here, simply fled. Babies lingered alone until they were discharged to foster care. Volunteers held and fed them. Nurses rocked them while they did their charts.

Tom and I could not help but perform a grim accounting as we surveyed the room. All of the other babies were bigger. But ours didn't shudder with seizures or wear a bandage on her head. She had all her parts, all her chromosomes.

Of the parents, we were among the privileged few. We had each other. We had good jobs. We could take time off. We lived nearby. We spoke English. We were sober.

Other couples conferred with translators, straining to decipher the language, the science, the odds. Fathers stumbled in after babies who had been helicoptered to the hospital roof. Some dads came dressed for the office or the golf course, interrupted by unfathomable events. They looked as though they'd just woken up, perhaps wondering if this were real. The fathers wore the same stunned faces. The mothers just looked pale and infinitely sad.

We saw a couple no older than sixteen, surrounded by family and balloons. The boy looked barely old enough to shave. We expected him to disappear, but he came back day after day in his white undershirt and too-big shorts. "Do you have any questions?" the doctors asked. He just shook his head.

Every life in the pod would be changed in some way, forever, including ours.

In the first five days, I slept maybe five hours. I didn't shower. The simple act of standing next to her incubator made me dizzy, so Tom would push a chair under me and I would lean on the lid and look down at her, my breath condensing on the plastic. The vomit stayed crusted in my hair. The capillaries under my eyes were busted from crying.

We were assigned a social worker and a patient advocate. We didn't need drug counseling, gas money, or a room at the Ronald McDonald House. But in those first days, we were summoned downstairs to meet with a financial specialist to sort out who was going to pay for all of this.

On the way there, I panicked. Clearly, we were lucky, but we weren't rich. I was working at a newspaper reeling from the upheaval in the industry, a newspaper that won Pulitzer Prizes but also wrestled with layoffs and buyouts. My pay had been cut twice. The extra money Tom made at Indiana University went to his Bloomington apartment and his Southwest Airlines commute.

The financial specialist was sweet and calm, but when we sat down at her desk, I gripped Tom's arm. I knew that medical disasters like this cost people their homes, their careers, their retirements, their marriages. I was paralyzed by the fear that if our daughter lived, she'd come home to a ruin of the family that had created her. This was before Obamacare, and most insurance plans, including the one at the newspaper, had lifetime caps. We had switched to the IU plan, because it was cheaper, but I couldn't remember anything about what it covered. Babies born this young almost always exceeded $1 million in medical expenses. If she lived, there would be deductibles, therapies, maybe even long-term care.

"You can't think about that right now," the specialist said. Ability to pay did not determine who got treatment and who did not. Most of the babies ended up on Medicaid. I was nearly hyperventilating when she said, "Well, this is amazing news."

She swiveled toward us in her chair. "It's only going to cost you four hundred dollars."

That was the co-pay for our baby's hospitalization. Everything that happened to her until she was discharged would be covered by Blue Cross Blue Shield. We had one of the best private insurance plans she'd seen in a long time. There would be plenty of expenses later, but I didn't hear much from that point forward.

After that ordeal, the people in charge of birth certificates began hounding me at all hours. They wanted a name and they by God wanted it now. Tom and I had been in such collision over names that we'd tabled the discussion until the third trimester. It still wasn't the third trimester, but the Name Police didn't care. They came to my room in the middle of the night, leaving behind a baby name book. They stalked me, wielding blank forms. At one point, with my gut freshly stapled shut, I actually tried to outrun one.

The card on the foot of her incubator said, simply, FRENCH, BABY GIRL and gave her birth weight: 570 grams. I've eaten burritos at Chipotle bigger than that.

I couldn't summon the will to care about the name problem. She could start kindergarten as Baby Girl French. Right now we had larger concerns. The biggest fear was intraventricular hemorrhage: bleeding in the brain. Vessels could burst from the stress of delivery or a surge in blood pressure. Blood could clot, causing pressure to build. Brain tissue could die, destroying the capacity for movement, language, learning. A bad enough brain bleed would mean taking her off life support.

In times of stress, the body diverts blood to the brain and heart first, the gut last. A lack of circulation could make her belly distend and blacken. Her intestines could wither, poisoning her from the inside.

The ventilator kept her alive, but the force of it stretched her tiny air sacs, scarring her lungs. A surge in pressure—from aggressive resuscitation, for example—could burst the air sacs. Too much pressure in the blood vessels could fill the lungs with blood, drowning her.

Antibiotics to ward off infection could shut down the kidneys. Oxygen to keep her alive could make her blind. Narcotics to keep her comfortable could make her an addict.

Our nurse warned us to keep our hopes in check.

"Never trust a preemie," she said.

None of our friends knew what kind of card to send. Were we celebrating or grieving? Even we didn't know.

"Congratulations!" people said, but that didn't seem quite right.

Friends and co-workers filled our freezer with cannelloni and lasagna. They held back the baby gifts they'd bought, not knowing if they would ever be used. Everyone, it seemed, knew somebody who knew somebody who was born at one pound and went on to have a remarkable life. Tom's co-worker's wife. A waitress's father. Without exception, it seemed, these babies were tucked into shoe boxes and kept warm by the oven.

"When can you take her home?" people asked, and it always stung.

Ours wasn't the world's smallest baby. Babies weighing just over nine ounces have survived, and ours weighed more than twice that. But gestational age, not birth weight, was the key predictor of how a baby would do. Our baby was born so early, some hospitals would have refused to save her. If she had come one week earlier, All Children's would have declined to try. In most countries, resuscitation would have been impossible. In others, it would have been all but forbidden.

When she was four days old, I was discharged. Tom pushed me out in a wheelchair, no baby in my arms, no balloons. I cried on the curb.

"It's a miracle," people would say. I'd thank them and grind my teeth and think, *Ask me in a year if it's a miracle.*

Tom

Kelley had finally drifted off, tossing and turning, her face tight with worry. I was too charged up to sleep, both terrified and giddy. I wanted to make sure our days-old daughter was still alive. I wanted to pretend that she would never die. So I went to the NICU and stood by her incubator and tried to accept the impossible.

She had inherited her mother's fierceness. It wasn't scientifically feasible, since she carried none of Kelley's DNA, but somehow it was true. The nurses were already talking about how formidable she was. When one of the techs performed an echocardiogram on her, passing the ultrasound wand over her sunken chest, her miniature hand reached up and seized the wand. The tech tried to pull it away, but the baby wouldn't let go.

"Man," said the tech. "She's strong."

My daughter's arm was as thin as a pencil and had no fat, no tone, no muscles to speak of. Yet she was playing tug-of-war with someone more than a hundred times her size.

The battle over naming her raged on. I had rejected Kelley's suggestion of Sawyer, and she had dismissed my nominations, starting with Elizabeth and Miranda and Katharine. Grandmother names, she called them. For the moment, we just called her Peanut, or Tater, short for Tater Tot.

As I stood there that night, I thought I saw her eyes fluttering behind her eyelids. I had read that micro-preemies have REMs, and I wondered what she could be dreaming about without ever having seen a single thing. Probably she relied on the other senses, imagining herself floating back in the womb, warm and secure, hearing the thump of her mother's heartbeat and the muffled rhythms of her voice. She was edging into consciousness. Everything about her seemed mysterious and otherworldly. Just watching her breathe made me happy.

I was in the throes of an odd delusion. Intellectually I recognized the perils my baby faced. But I had fallen in love with this child, and the idea that she could be taken from me and from her mother, after all we had been through, was too cruel to accept. So I concocted a gauzy layer of fiction. Like my daughter, I was temporarily blind.

The notion that I was watching her breathe was a lie. She was not breathing. A machine was breathing for her. I found it easy to gloss over this distinction. I was not yet strong enough to contemplate the true nature of this strange and sealed-off place, filled with patients so small they had no business being alive, human beings not yet fully human, swaddled in artificial darkness and cradled by machines.

Kelley saw it. Maybe she saw it too well. She was having nightmares and finding it difficult to get out of bed. She wanted to be optimistic, but the reality of the odds kept tipping her toward paralyzing despair. She found it intensely painful to enter the NICU. Every time she listened to the doctors, the things they said made her want to run.

I could not stay away from the pod. There was a purity to it that I found unexpectedly invigorating. I had already made arrangements for other professors to take over my journalism classes in Indiana until the semester ended. For now, I was done with the weekly commutes. No more airports, no more editing students' drafts on planes. I was free to focus entirely on Kelley and the baby. I had a mission, and the urgency of it trumped my usual anxieties.

It was close to midnight. Nat and Sam had booked their flights to come see the baby that weekend, and my sister Brooke was driving down from Atlanta. I couldn't wait for them all to meet her, and I was sure they would help us figure out what to call her. A real name, I told myself, would protect her. Another illusion.

I pulled back a corner of the quilt and leaned against the top of the incubator and studied her fingers, so long and delicate, and the curl of her toes, and her folds of extra skin, waiting to fill out as she grew. Her shoulders were still feathered with lanugo, the fine hair that grows in the womb and then falls out shortly after birth. Even that I found gorgeous.

The young nurse assigned to her that night told me her weight was dropping a little, but that was normal.

"Everything's good," she said before hurrying away to check on her other patients.

The euphoria was rising in me again. The certainty that our daughter would be fine.

I hadn't confessed my delusion to Kelley or anyone else, because I didn't want to jinx it and because I knew that if I heard myself say such things out loud, the lies I was telling myself would lose their power. As each day passed, my secret faith in our baby's survival grew stronger. If I believed it fervently enough, maybe it would come true.

By now I had learned that the nurses were superstitious and did not like to tempt fate by saying the unit was quiet. The Q-word, they called it, and they frowned when anyone uttered it out loud. But at that hour, there was no other way to describe Six South. The lights had been dimmed, but this end of the pod was swimming in a soft orange glow coming from a wall of windows that faced westward toward Tropicana Field. Baseball season was starting, and the Tampa Bay Rays had beaten the Minnesota Twins that night on a tenth-inning home run. Whenever the Rays won at home, the Trop's dome glowed orange. From a distance, the oval looked like a shimmering mother ship, floating just above the rooftops. I stared transfixed, caught off guard by this reminder that baseball games were still being played and that fans were still buying hot dogs for their kids and yelling at the umps and that the world was still spinning.

Almost all of the babies appeared to be sleeping inside their cocoons. I heard a nurse talking to one, telling him he needed to behave, and it made me smile.

I decided to memorize the names of all the nurses and the techs and the doctors, to gather whatever intel I could about their kids or their dogs, their favorite TV shows, anything that might allow me to strike up a conversation. In my iPad I was tapping out notes and making charts and cataloging characteristics to help me keep them straight.

Dr. Eeyore and Dr. Yoda were easy. But there were hundreds of other staff members on the floor. This respiratory tech, I noted, had a southern accent. Another was a belly dancer in her spare time and was a good listener. The nurse next to us had a young son who thought he wanted to be a writer. The nurse at the other end of the pod had the gruff voice of a prison matron, but when she changed a baby's diaper, she dissolved into sweetness, cooing and cajoling. I kept expecting her to pull a Brach's caramel out of her pocket and pop it into a preemie's mouth. Another wore a sparkly hair band and talked in an extra-perky voice, like an overcaffeinated cheerleader. She turned up the bubble voice when she spoke to parents, especially dads, but talked like a normal person with her co-workers.

I pushed myself to say hello to them all, to make eye contact and smile. I was cultivating the persona of the harmless dad—unobtrusive, nonconfrontational, eager to help. I was in fact all of those things. But the persona masked my calculated attempts to eke out an advantage for my daughter. I recognized that there was something unseemly in my plotting, but I didn't care. Once we got past our first week in the NICU and everything settled down, I would bake dozens of chocolate chip cookies and bring in one heaping plate for the day shift and another for the night shift. I was determined to charm the entire floor.

"Once they get to know us, and get to know our baby, maybe they'll pay closer attention," I told Kelley. "If something goes wrong, maybe they'll run a little faster."

Peanut was squeezing my finger again. Was she awake now, or just reacting in her sleep? I didn't know if she was scared or in pain. Whatever she was experiencing inside the darkness, I wanted her to know that she had me and her mother and two big brothers, and that someday soon she would open her eyes, and the light would fill the world, and she would see our faces and know she was ours. The tube would come out, and she would be able to cry and tell us when she hurt, and before she knew it, she would be big enough for us to take her home, where her real life would begin.

The ventilator breathed in and out, mocking me.

Kelley

Things that weigh 570 grams:

1. A six-week-old kitten
2. A Smith & Wesson LadySmith double-action .38 special revolver
3. A bottle of Gatorade
4. A raw bone-in rib eye
5. The left lung of an adult human female
6. The amount of breast milk an eight-pound baby drinks in one day
7. $2.28 in pennies
8. An adult eastern gray squirrel

Tom

We sought escape wherever we could: the hospital cafeteria, the sixth-floor lounge, where we watched old episodes of *Law & Order*. One afternoon I went to Publix, just so I could remember what it was like to push a grocery cart. I was in the produce section, hunting for a decent bag of green grapes, when I heard the alarm from the baby's monitor, warning that her oxygen saturation was dropping. I looked up to check the aqua-blue number and was starting to wonder where the nurse had gone when I realized that the only thing above me were fluorescent lights. The alarm stopped. Seconds later, it started again. This time I ignored it until all I could hear were the wheels of the cart jangling across the linoleum.

I pushed on, trying not to think about the hospital. But when I came to the baking aisle, my hand reached for a small bag of sugar. I placed it in my palm, lifting it up and down, gauging the lightness of it. One pound was nothing. One pound could be poured away in an instant. The other shoppers pushed their carts around me, pretending they did not see the strange man crying over the sugar.

Kelley

The baby was the baton, passed from nurse to nurse every twelve hours. The morning doctor was not the night doctor. The weekday doctor was off on weekends. The doctor in charge rotated every three weeks. The neonatologist asked for the nephrologist, who sent a resident. They were a blur. Their names didn't matter. Tom fussed with his notebooks and charts.

People kept telling us that parents counted here. Someone had to keep track of things. The computerized charting system couldn't replace human concentration and intuition. We were supposed to stand guard, to keep watch. But for what?

The alarm sounded and quieted. The baby twitched and scowled, and mostly slept.

We were advised to identify a great nurse and ask that person to be our daughter's primary caretaker. If she agreed — most of the nurses were women — she would take care of our baby whenever she worked. She would bring consistency to a fragmented operation. She would be our sounding board and our interpreter.

How would we find such a person? There were so many nurses. Day shift and night. Tom started asking around. Nurses were reluctant to single out each other, but we could tell a little by the things not said. Some nurses were better with parents than babies, we were told. We needed someone who could do it all.

A patient-care representative whispered to Tom that Tracy Hullett was the best in the unit. We knew who she was, because she had already taken care of Peanut once or twice. We began to study her while she worked.

Tracy moved quietly, in the background, and was hard to read. She had a wicked smile, a voice that remained calm when every alarm was sounding. She had worked at All Children's forever and remembered everything that had ever gone wrong or ever gone right on the sixth floor. She was no one's boss, but she helped hold the unit together. She treated everyone with respect, including the sweet Jamaican woman who mopped the floor early every morning.

"Hi, Mary," Tracy would say, patting her on the shoulder as she slipped by. "How you doing?"

Some of the other nurses wore scrubs decorated with teddy bears or Tweety Bird. Tracy's were adorned with cats from outer space and monkeys performing downward-facing dog. She had a thing about zebra stripes and wore them on her clogs. She was meticulous but had a gift for improvisation. She hemmed her pants with staples. She was sharp-edged and sardonic and entertained us with disaster stories from her love life, including the time she dumped a guy because he was stupid enough to woo her with carnations. I nodded sympathetically while Tom shook his head on behalf of men everywhere.

Tracy didn't have kids of her own and didn't want them. She joked that she only liked the tiny babies.

"I lose interest in them once they cut teeth."

That was fine with us. We wanted her to save our baby's life, not teach her to water-ski. Tracy had six rescued cats—like me, she had a soft spot for wounded things. She moved so stealthily, she came to remind us of a cat. She had a gift for invisibility and could disappear without anyone noticing, then show up again precisely when she was needed. Everything about her declared her absolute proficiency. In just two days of watching her work, I had learned that she was a master of small details. Our daughter's diaper was the size of a pack of Trident, and yet Tracy could change it in an instant without a single tug on the wires. When she replaced the dressings that held the tubes in place, she would touch her fingers to the sticky side of the tape, weakening the glue so it wouldn't tear skin.

Some of the nurses did not talk much to their patients; others soothed them with baby talk. Tracy spoke to Peanut as though the baby understood everything happening around her. When the baby was hitting or kicking, Tracy knew how to calm her down.

"Now listen, young lady," Tracy told her. "I've been wrestling preemies for a long time, and I'm not afraid of you."

Then, in response, she would slip into the imagined voice of our baby: "Tracy, I thought we were friends."

No one intimidated Tracy. One morning, when a doctor ordered a barrage of blood tests, we watched her calmly pick up a phone to remind him that our daughter had a little more than an ounce of blood in her entire body.

"This baby doesn't have that much blood to give," Tracy said. "You're going to have to decide which tests you want the most."

She had a steady, no-nonsense Hoosier sensibility, which drew in Tom immediately. We were nervous about touching the baby, so she showed us how to do it without setting off any alarms. The baby's skin was so new and the nerves so close to the surface that stroking rankled her. She liked firm, steady pressure that made her feel secure, as in the womb. We'd cup one hand around her head and the other around her feet. We could feel the soft spots throbbing in her skull.

Tracy would gently turn her each time she tucked her in, so the baby's soft head wouldn't flatten on the sides. It was an effect common in preemies that the nurses called toaster head. Once I learned about toaster heads I saw them everywhere. In the elevator. In the grocery. *Preemie!* I'd think, proud of my new diagnostic abilities. I wanted my baby to be brilliant and have a nice round head like Charlie Brown, but mostly I wanted her to live. If she ended up with a head like a kitchen appliance, well, kids look so great in hats.

I shared every one of these crazed thoughts with Tracy, and she didn't appear to judge me. We were a great fit.

I was too nervous to ask her. I have the social skills of a tree stump, so I made Tom do it. He caught Tracy one morning, early, as she walked away from another baby's incubator. She saw him coming. I watched as the two of them stood frozen in the middle of the pod. I could tell he was fumbling. Tracy looked away, muttered something, then hurried off.

"She said she wasn't sure she had time," Tom reported when he came back. She had too many other duties on the floor. The charge nurse needed her on a catheter team and on the IV burn team.

I gave him a look, pressing for more.

"She said she'd think about it."

Tom

Make-believe came easily then. We anesthetized ourselves with the rituals of new parenthood. We wandered the baby aisles at Target, luxuriating in the narcotic haze of soft pinks and yellows and blues. We were so hungry for a fix of normalcy that we couldn't resist throwing a few items into our cart. Another book of baby names to help us narrow in on a final pick; extra-soft blankets that made us feel as though we were decorating her nursery at home instead of brightening up the coffin-shaped plastic box. A small stuffed giraffe that played rain sounds to drown out the ventilator's mechanical hiss.

With every day, my secret faith in her indestructibility deepened. I hung on every word at morning rounds, when the medical team assembled and delivered their daily assessment. I loved the rolling pageantry, the way the neonatologist led the procession by pushing forward her big computer tricked out on a tall tray with wheels, so she could glide and pivot, remaining standing through it all as her fingers marched across the keyboard, summoning the latest X-rays and ultrasounds, updates on our baby's blood gases and her white blood count and her lipids, the missives from cardiology and nephrology and neurology. I took comfort in all those "ologies," the implication of a sprawling network buried somewhere in the lower floors of the hospital. I imagined an army of doctors toiling in soundproof labs, bent over electron microscopes and whirring centrifuges, and calculated their centuries of collective expertise.

I loved the way the team opened each morning's rounds with the same ceremonial words. "Baby Girl French, day of life four," or five or six. I reveled in the sober, flat tone of the team's assessments, the nodding and conferring, the clearing of throats, the recommendations and counter-recommendations, the cautious estimates of risk and reward, as though we were convened at the Pentagon. I did not understand their jargon, the rush of their acronyms and allusions. The impenetrability of their language seemed to imbue them with a higher power. I felt it in the syncopated rhythms of their UAC and TPN and RBC transfusions, in the restorative aura of their vitamin A protocols and their crits and clotting studies, the endless doses of life-giving ampicillin and gentamicin and fentanyl and Zosyn, the beguiling mysteries of their tidal volumes and coagulopathy. The more incomprehensible their pronouncements, the more I believed these people were our salvation.

The smallest details of the hospital filled me with irrational wonder. When the elevators came alive with the recorded voices of the children, I smiled, knowing those kids had once been patients. Now they sounded so strong and happy! A grand piano waited in the lobby, and I would sometimes see one of the doctors, a surgeon who specialized in pediatric plastic surgery, leaning over the keyboard, regaling visitors with soaring melodies. This surgeon was known for his kindness and skill, and when I heard him playing, my mind would catapult forward to the day when our daughter would be released from the NICU and we would pause on our way out so she could sit beside him on the piano bench. He would tap out something sweet for her, something that made her giggle, and she would plink the keys with her tiny fingers.

Kelley and I found solace in the stream of friends and family who came to meet our daughter. Sam, sick with bronchitis, was forced to cancel his flight because he could not risk making the baby sick. Nat arrived late that Thursday night. He had already seen a picture of the baby connected to all the wires and tubes, but it wasn't until he saw me waiting for him at the airport, my face lined with exhaustion, that he realized things were so serious. Later, he told me it was the first time he'd ever seen me looking unsure of anything.

In the NICU the next morning, Nat reached inside the incubator and opened his palm above his sister's body. Curled on her side, she was exactly the size of his hand.

My sister Brooke arrived that evening. We wanted to get to the NICU early Saturday so we could be there for the start of the day shift. Kelley was in bad shape and didn't want to get out of bed. It was her first morning after being discharged, and she couldn't stand the quiet. Just the idea of walking by the healthy-baby nursery again was too much for her. She knew we needed to get to the hospital but hated being left alone in the empty house. I tried to talk to her, but she turned her back to me.

"I'll be fine," she said. "Just go in."

Driving toward the hospital, I told Brooke how beautiful the baby was and how well she was doing.

"Not many parents get to see their child so soon," I said. "They don't get to see what their baby looks like at this point.

But we do. We can talk to her and watch her developing, right in front of our eyes."

If Brooke thought it was strange to hear her brother gushing, she did not say so.

Up on the sixth floor, I led her to Bed 692. I was already addicted to watching visitors' faces when they saw the baby for the first time. First came the slap of shock, then comprehension deepening into acceptance. After a few minutes, when they saw that she was breathing and moving and not about to expire in front of them, they relaxed. Slowly their faces blossomed as they realized they were seeing something they had never seen before, something terrifying and wondrous, something undeniably sacred.

Brooke was steady, but her eyes brimmed. Then she broke, beaming and crying and asking a dozen questions.

The nurse that day was Jackie, who reminded me of a sassy grandmother. On the baby's head she had nestled a crocheted cap. Beneath the baby she had spread a crocheted blanket of the same pastel pattern. Over the incubator she had draped a crocheted afghan. It was essential, she said, that my daughter matched.

"I may not be a lady," Jackie told us with a wink. "But she is."

Brooke and I loved her, and we were relieved when she assured us that the baby was stable. I occupied myself by studying the incubators that surrounded us. We weren't allowed to walk up to look at the babies inside. Kelley had tried it and been stopped by a nurse quoting privacy regulations. And although there was no rule against talking with other parents, the idea of it felt awkward. They were encased so tightly in their own sorrows that they seemed out of reach. It was like riding a crowded subway in New York. We were all on top of one another but exiled in our own worlds.

As we sat there, Brooke and I realized something was happening with the baby in 695, the incubator across from ours. One moment everything was quiet, then a nurse hurried up and opened the top of the incubator, and then one of the neonatologists was called over, and then more nurses. I don't remember anyone telling us we needed to leave, but their urgency made it obvious that they needed to focus without being watched.

When we took Kelley to lunch, she picked at her food. I tried to draw her out, kissing her cheek. She would rally for a second, then drift away.

That afternoon, Jennifer joined us at the hospital, and we all turned our attention to picking a name. We couldn't put it off any longer. The card taped to the front of her incubator still referred to her only as FRENCH, BABY GIRL, as though a stork had flown her over from Marseilles. As though she were wearing a tiny beret.

Momentum was building toward Juniper. Our only reservation was that we didn't want to make her sound like one of Frank Zappa's grandchildren. My sister, an elementary-school teacher, had seen her share of crazy kid names: Thalo, Blaze, Dante, Riles, 2dayy. She assured us that our pick fell on the respectable side of that line.

"I know three Junipers," Jennifer offered. "They're all my dirty hippie friends, but still."

"Juniper, then," Kelley said. She liked that Juniper and Jennifer came from the same root word and that they'd been linked in that Donovan song, riding that dappled mare.

"Ju-ni-per," I said, sounding it out. "Junebug. Junie-june."

I could hear it bouncing playfully off her tongue at age six when she introduced herself on the playground while hanging from the monkey bars. I saw it rippling across the face of the ten-year-old boy who finally worked up the courage to approach her under the disco-ball lights at the roller rink. Poor kid. He'd be so flustered, he'd fall on his ass and watch her skate away without a backward glance. Time hurtled forward, and I felt the Old Testament heft of the name when she stormed into the courtroom in her flowing black robe.

"All rise!" the bailiff would boom. "Circuit Court is now in session. The Honorable Juniper A. French presiding."

We celebrated our choice with a gelato run downtown. The sun was disappearing over the Gulf, a breeze playing through the leaves of the massive banyans across the street. Children were climbing in the trees' roots and reaching up to run their fingertips through tendrils of Spanish moss.

Kelley was still quiet, but Brooke and I laughed and hooted and teetered along the sidewalk with our arms thrown over each other's shoulders, singing like drunken idiots. If the nurses had heard me, they would have scolded me back to reality.

Back in the NICU, we told the nurses we had settled on a name. Brooke and I could not help looking over at 695. It was empty, as was 696, which had been occupied earlier in the day by a squirming baby. Both monitors were turned off, and the bedding was rolled up.

"What happened to six ninety-five and six ninety-six?" I asked one of the nurses, trying to sound casual. "Where did they go?"

She told me that the patient in 696 was doing so well that they'd transferred her to another unit. She said nothing about 695 and quickly walked away.

I froze. In that moment, I began to understand that Six

135

South floated in a cloud of randomness. The baby in 695 had done nothing wrong. Maybe Death simply liked to play tag. Maybe Death was smiling at Juniper and getting ready to tap her on the shoulder.

Kelley closed her eyes and chanted under her breath.

"Oh God, oh God, oh God, oh…"

Kelley

Day and night, I was anchored to the breast pump, a massive hospital-grade industrial model that might as well have been a dungeon wall. I plugged it in next to the bed and filled a shelf with little plastic bottles with yellow caps, extra tubing, and the weird plastic funnels I was supposed to hold to my chest. My body still wasn't working right, so what should have taken fifteen minutes took hours. I'd end up with a few drops, maybe. The pump groaned and heaved like an old woman—an old woman who had probably nursed a dozen fat babies with her pendulous breasts—and in my head I heard it mocking me.

You're pathetic.

You're pathetic.

You're pathetic.

It would be simplistic to say I felt like a dairy cow. Dairy cows produced milk. I had failed. I'd failed to conceive, failed to carry a baby to term, now I was failing to feed my barely formed daughter. If I were livestock, I'd be culled from the herd.

No one had to remind me that this was important. Breast milk killed everything from *E. coli* to cholera. It brimmed with antibodies. If I so much as looked at a sick person, the lactation consultants assured me, my boobs would cue up a protective potion.

You're pathetic.

You're pathetic.

I couldn't pump at the hospital, though they provided every convenience and even a reward system. Turn in any amount of milk to the Milk Depot, and receive a coupon from the hospital cafeteria for all the pudding and rotisserie chicken you could carry.

Pumping at the hospital meant spending those hours in a tiny, windowless room, with a poster of a wrinkled, hairy-faced preemie on the wall. In that room I was just close enough to my baby to feel more gravely the weight of my failure. It still felt like every hour could be her last, so every hour in that room was a loss. Pumping at her bedside was an option, but an absurd one, given that she shared a room with other babies, other families, the constant interruption of doctors, nurses, nurse practitioners, respiratory therapists, phlebotomists, patient-care assistants, social workers.

The next day, I stayed home, moored to the pump, trying to kick-start my body into behaving. I felt uneasy, almost panicky, in a way I couldn't explain. When Tom woke up, I asked him to call the NICU, because I was afraid to dial the phone myself. He supplied our patient access code—5149—to Jackie, our nurse again that day. Jackie said cheerfully that Juniper was fine. She was wearing a pink hat and resting on a pink blanket. But the feeling didn't go away. That afternoon, I asked Tom to call again. She was still fine. Maybe it was my guilt, but I wasn't convinced.

That evening, as I packed the mostly empty milk bottles to

take to the NICU, a young nurse named Whitney Hoertz started her shift at six. She told us later that she had looked at the monitors and the chart. All good. She looked at the results of that afternoon's chest X-ray. All good. Then she looked at the baby.

Juniper's belly looked a little dark, maybe, but it could be hard to tell in the light. Whitney got out a measuring tape and wrapped it under and around her. Her belly measured eighteen centimeters—it had grown by one and a half centimeters since that morning. That was not good. She had learned in nursing school about a fearsome condition called necrotizing enterocolitis, which kills many of the tiniest babies. Whitney had never seen it herself, but she knew a swollen abdomen was one of the first signs. She called a doctor, who called for an X-ray.

We were arriving at the hospital when my cell phone rang. Whitney's hunch had been right. Juniper's intestine had ruptured. The doctors called it a perf, as in perforation, which sounds so fixable, something you could patch like a bicycle tire. Air and stool were spilling and collecting in her abdomen, flooding it with bacteria. This was the very calamity I'd hoped to inoculate her against by pumping the lousy milk. Studies were clear that breast milk was the best defense against this, but my shortage had meant she'd received some formula, too. I'd failed again.

"How soon can you be here?" the doctor asked.

"We're parking," I said. "We'll be there in five."

We rushed through the hospital's main doors and up to the NICU to find a gathering at her bedside. The lid was off the incubator, and she lay there, distended and subdued. Her body hadn't deteriorated to the point that the monitors would register any trouble. Whitney's hunch had been the only warning.

We had never seen her so clearly, so close, as we did now. Her face was turned to the side, and I could see that her head was still soft, that it reshaped itself each time she was turned. It was flattish on the sides. Her hair was so dark it looked wet. We each held her hands in our fingertips for a second.

Someone presented a consent form. I signed without reading. Then we were ushered out.

The surgeons inserted a drain, like a soft drinking straw, to wick away the gunk in her belly. All we could do was wait to see if she healed, or if infection took her down, or if her intestines died off. It was a good thing she'd been getting breast milk, they said. Maybe it would help.

We struggled to find the right thing to say to the twenty-eight-year-old nurse who had seen what the monitors could not.

"Whitney," Tom said. "Whitney..."

"I know," she said. "I don't know what would've happened either."

We wanted to spend the night by Juniper's side, so while the surgeons worked, we dashed home to let out the dog. Tom lingered over the bookshelves in the office and emerged carrying the first volume of the *Harry Potter* series, the hardcover edition.

"Are you sure she's ready for that?" I asked him delicately. "How about something a little lighter? You know, like *Goodnight Moon*?"

I knew Tom saw the world through the lens of story. But I

didn't know why he'd chosen *Harry Potter*. She wouldn't understand a word of it. I just knew that the choice was part of the story he was writing about himself, about the kind of dad he was to her in that moment.

By now it was midnight. As we pulled off the interstate, we could see the lights of the hospital. As always, our eyes went to the sixth floor.

"I just don't want her to be alone," Tom said. "I want her to know she is not alone."

When we arrived, he pulled up a stool beside the incubator and opened the book.

" 'Chapter One,' " he began. " 'The Boy Who Lived.' "

It was an act of faith, I suppose, choosing the first book in a series that totaled more than four thousand pages. I knew he intended to read the entire thing, all seven books, even if it took him seven years. I hoped he would get to read them again someday when she could really understand. I also knew this might be his only chance.

We watched the numbers flash on the monitor. The green number for the heart rate. The white number for her breathing. The blue number for the oxygen saturation in her blood. Those numbers were mesmerizing. I stared at them, not sleeping, as the floor grew quiet and the windows grew dark.

Whitney brought me a blanket. I sank into a chair for the night and listened to Tom reading, fighting tears, reading again. The book tells the story of a baby who survived an attack by the most powerful evil in the world. He survived because his mother stood by his crib and protected him with her life. Tom fell asleep slumped against the incubator, using the book as a pillow.

The next morning, I awoke to find that he'd moved to the chair next to me. Except for his snoring, the NICU was so quiet, which seemed odd. A baby's life could hang on a matter of minutes or hours. A crisis could happen at any time of day or night. Why should there be fewer doctors on guard, just because it was 5:00 a.m.? I was relieved to see the sky lighten outside the windows, like a curtain lifting. Soon more doctors would arrive, and surgeons and specialists and, I imagined, someone with some goddamn answers. I pictured them in their white coats, astride cavalry horses.

Around six, a technician rolled a portable ultrasound machine to Juniper's bedside. He raised the lid and cradled her head in one hand. With the other hand he placed the ultrasound wand against the wide, pulsing fontanelle. My heart hit my throat, and I nudged Tom awake.

This was the test that would show us whether she had suffered bleeding in her brain. I'd been too upset about her belly to remember that it was scheduled for today, her sixth day of life. If it showed a massive bleed, the prognosis could mean severe and permanent disability. That, combined with the life-threatening rupture in her belly and everything else, would mean we would take her off life support, because how much insult could a one-pound baby take?

Most of the tiniest babies in the NICU don't die on their own. They are babies who would have died without intervention. So here, they die by decision. They are taken off life support by agreement of their parents and doctors, when the suffering becomes too great and the prognosis becomes too grim.

This exam, which I'd completely forgotten, would go a long

way toward determining whether Juniper was allowed to continue to fight.

I tried to divine some meaning from the image on the monitor. I saw the gray expanse of her brain and, inside it, two pools of black. I knew from the many ultrasounds during my pregnancy that black meant fluid. They looked like oil spills.

Blood? The technician, I knew, would tell us nothing.

I whispered to Tom, "Is fluid black?"

"I don't know, sweetie," he said, taking in the machine, the tech, the monitor. "Let's not jump to conclusions."

I saw the tech capture a few images, and then he wheeled his cart away.

For the next few hours, Tom fumbled with his iPad, reading the *Huffington Post* and the *New York Times,* and in me a frustration simmered. How could he be such a slave to current events? For three days, tornadoes had been ripping apart the southern United States, killing dozens of people, but there was no room in me for other people's misery. Did he not understand that our lives were splintering? On my iPad, I Googled "ultrasound of brain."

I tried to reconcile the images I found with what I'd seen on the monitor. Apparently, we all have fluid in our heads. It bathes and cushions the brain. If we didn't have cavities in there, our heads would be too heavy for our necks. I had no idea, though, if the black pools I'd seen were normal.

More hours rolled by. Two or three, I don't know how many. Tom and I were still cramped and bleary in the chairs next to the incubator when a small, slow-moving battalion came rolling through the unit. Morning rounds.

The cavalry.

At the center of the group, Dr. Fauzia Shakeel wore the granite stare I so needed to see. With her long white coat and shiny dark hair, she looked like she could defend our baby against whatever came: bacteria, viruses, dark magic. The members of her entourage flipped through charts, kept their backs straight. Clearly, no one wanted to get caught unprepared.

Diane, the nurse practitioner, read from the chart. "This is Juniper French, day of life six, she weighs six hundred grams, up forty from yesterday." She bristled under Dr. Shakeel's firm command. Just to be safe, I scrambled out of the chair to my feet.

Dr. Shakeel already knew what was in the chart, I could tell. She had read it herself ahead of time. This made me love her.

Worsening blood gases...metabolic acidosis...Penrose draining blood-tinged fluid...

Dr. Shakeel glanced at us. I chewed maniacally on a cuticle.

The computer showed a new report from radiology that morning.

Dr. Shakeel looked up from the monitor, softened, and smiled.

"Her head is fine," she said.

Tom caught me as I fell.

That day we found by her incubator a worn hardcover edition of *Field Book of American Trees and Shrubs*. We never figured out who left it there, but we did learn that junipers are hardy. We took this as a good omen.

Our daughter was still horribly sick. The ventilator had strained the air sacs in her lungs, so the doctors put her on a gentler oscillating machine that made her whole body vibrate.

They called it the hi-fi. Watching her chest, we saw no rhythmic rise and fall, no visual cue that she was a living, breathing person. Just a bizarre, full-body shudder.

The ventilator was as big and noisy as a washing machine full of rocks. We hated it for crowding us out of the narrow space beside her bed, for making her appear a little less human, for making us think about her sheer fragility. At rounds a couple of days later, the doctor explained that most babies her size would have chronic lung disease all their lives.

"She probably won't run a marathon," he said. It sounded like a line he had used many times, and it stung more than I would have expected. I wasn't ready to concede any corner of Juniper's future. Of course I knew she could die. I ricocheted between the disappointment that she might not run a marathon and the possibility that she might not ever walk. I had no equilibrium.

No one discussed it, but when the brain scan came back clean, we had cleared a threshold. I wish I had recognized it then, because I was still spinning, grasping for any foothold on our future. But at that moment, while she still faced death or an array of handicaps beyond our control, the test suggested her brain could be okay. She might someday laugh, sing, and call me Mom.

The day she'd been born, we could have let her die, and no one would have judged us. Now it would be much harder to take her off life support. Our moral obligation had grown heavier.

There's a phrase in neonatology: "waiting to declare." Doctors say they stabilize the baby at birth and then wait for them to declare themselves—their intentions and their will—by either improving or deteriorating.

Juniper

Juniper was no longer a fetus. She had crossed into person-hood. We had seen her and touched her and loved her. Day by day she cemented her stake in the world. We were still waiting for her to declare, but it was becoming harder and harder to turn back.

Tom

We drove back and forth to the hospital, barely noticing the stoplights or traffic. At home in bed, Kelley cried past midnight. I pulled her close, but it did no good. She stopped brushing her hair. People would call, and we could barely make out what they were saying. I forgot to shower or change my clothes, forgot to brush my teeth. I felt as though I were sliding out of the skin of the person I used to be.

"I don't know what we're supposed to do," I told Kelley one morning as she sat in bed, pumping her milk. "How do we get through this?"

She looked at me and shrugged.

Our friends mowed our lawn, checked our mail, kept restocking our fridge. Kelley's teammates from flyball rescued poor neglected Muppet and took her to their home to stay with them as long as needed. On the day Junebug was born, our friend Cherie, a sharp-eyed photographer from the paper, came to the NICU to take photos in case the baby didn't make it through the night. Later that afternoon, our friend Stephen showed up at the door of Kelley's hospital room, asking what he could do to help. Stephen has an almost supernatural calm, and it was all we could do not to collapse against him.

Roy Peter Clark, the older brother I never had, checked on me every day. I'd meet him at Banyan, our favorite coffeehouse, whenever I needed half an hour away. Sometimes we talked about the baby. Sometimes we talked about nothing—the depravity of Florida politics, the latest twist in *Game of Thrones,* the home runs Evan Longoria was knocking into the cheap seats at Tropicana Field.

Our friend Mike, a busy editor with three kids of his own, was always standing beside the incubator whenever we needed him. He brought us coffee, put his hand on our shoulders, and held us up. We had no idea if Junebug was going to make it, but we knew that Mike and Roy and Cherie and Stephen and so many others would never abandon us.

It was painful seeing a baby so small and in such distress. My father had a lifelong phobia of hospitals, and when he first saw his granddaughter sleeping in her nest of wires, he bolted to the nearest bathroom to throw up. He apologized to the nurses and to us over and over. He said his stomach had been bothering him all day. I believed him, but I had also seen the fear on his face. I knew he was shaken and wished there was something he could do. So he made a stab at hope.

"She's a miracle," he told me. "I know this is a hard time, but she's going to make it. I just know it."

A queasy feeling came over me as I heard my father echoing my secret mantra. Making things right with Kelley, all those years before, had saved me from my most destructive instincts. I knew that she needed me now. But if we didn't leave this hospital with Junebug in our arms, I could not see why Kelley would want me in her life.

*   *   *

Finally I was waking to the reality of the dangers facing our daughter. The disappearance of the baby in 695, the hole in Juniper's bowels, the possibility that her intestines were dying—all of it made it difficult to rationalize away death as theoretical. I understood now that we were stuck inside a limbo where each moment was suspended between life and no life, everything and nothing.

I couldn't just sit by the box and watch Junebug shudder and twitch. So every morning at dawn, when the nurses popped the top on her incubator and took her vitals and checked her color, I tried to make myself useful. I learned how to tuck a thermometer in her armpit without tearing the skin, even though Junebug fought me every time. I learned how to brush her hair without pressing her soft skull. How to swab the interior of her mouth with a lollipop-style sponge dipped in sterile water. Once a day, the nurses needed someone to lift her while they changed her blankets. The first time Tracy asked me to do it, I balked. What if the baby came apart in my hands?

Tracy coached me through it as if she were teaching me to defuse a bomb. I slipped my stubby fingers under my daughter and gathered the wires and tubes, then cupped her head in one hand and the rest of her body in the other, raising her a few inches. In my hands, she seemed to disappear. I could feel her bones shifting against my fingers.

"Good," Tracy said. "Just hold her there."

Tracy was around more and more. She never announced it, but we realized she'd decided to be our primary nurse after all. In her voice I heard a trace of a Hoosier accent. I had known and admired girls like her in high school—smart girls used to driving fast on back roads that cut through cornfields, armored in an unwavering sense of right and wrong, afraid of nothing and no one, with sharp tongues that could slice you in half if you got fresh, and not a lick of patience for anyone who put on airs. In my experience, these girls grew into women who quietly ran the world.

She told me she had never wanted to be a nurse, but her dad had pushed her into it. Years earlier, he had talked her mom out of nursing school, and he still felt guilty. Tracy did enroll in nursing school but quit for beauty college when she learned she would have to dissect a cat. Her father talked sense into her, and she dissected the cat.

"I'm glad he did that," I told her.

I wanted to pump my fist for Tracy's dad. It's too easy for fathers to feel wedged out of their children's lives. From pregnancy onward, the mother exists at the center of the universe, her body an ocean of safety, nourishment, comfort. Fathers can rub the mother's feet and make sure she eats and drive her to the doctor, but we are marooned from the baby. We direct our voice toward the mom's swelling belly and hope that whoever is inside will hear some garbled version of our words, mixing with the sound track of the mother's heartbeat and breath. When the child is born, she still believes she and her mother are one. The mother is a continent of completion. Her gravity is unbreakable.

The father is a bit player. He watches the mother nursing the baby and realizes he can never compete.

"You have two jobs now," another dad told me when Nat was born. "You're the mule, and you're the clown."

Junebug's early arrival, traumatic as it was, offered me a chance to help my daughter in a way few other men are ever granted. She was more vulnerable than any child I had ever known, but she was still a baby, and after a lifetime of practice, I had a few ideas on how to help. There was no handbook on how to bond with a micro-preemie, so I made it up. When someone from the lab came to draw more blood, I leaned close and told Junebug how brave she was. When a tech arrived to perform another echocardiogram, I sang "If I Only Had a Heart," the Tin Man's song from *The Wizard of Oz*. Her squinted eyes, on the verge now of prying open, turned in my direction. Maybe she saw an outline, maybe a blur. But I knew she could hear me, because whenever I read her another chapter from *The Sorcerer's Stone,* she grew quiet and still.

One of the therapists who worked with Junebug reminded me that the baby wouldn't understand what I was reading.

"It would be better if you just told her that you loved her," the therapist said. "Just keep telling her."

That was just it. Reading that book to my daughter was the best way I knew to show her what I felt. I had nothing against *Goodnight Moon.* When Nat and Sam were little, I had read it to them so many times that I could still recite many pages from memory, twenty years later. I wanted something I could read to Junebug for weeks, maybe months. The night I first opened *Harry Potter,* I knew she wasn't going to follow a word. But she wouldn't have understood *Goodnight Moon* either. She had never seen the moon, had no idea what a cow was, or a kitten or a brush or a bowl full of mush. All Juniper knew was the long night into which she had been born. That darkness was the entirety of her world, and it would have been easy for her to believe there was nothing beyond it.

I could not understand what it was inside this child,

this notion of a girl, that made her keep going. I wanted her to hear the joy and expectation in my voice, and the rhythms of J. K. Rowling's sentences, and the sense of something unfolding, something that hinted at all that waited outside the pod.

In our family, this copy of *Harry Potter* held special power. Nat and Sam and I had devoured it so many times we had lost the jacket. The purple and red of the cover was fading. The spine was warping. If I read these pages to Juniper, maybe she would sense our love for the story burning underneath the words. Maybe she would feel her brothers with her, even though they were a thousand miles away. I certainly felt the boys' presence every time I opened the book. Harry and Hermione had their spells. I needed to cast my own.

The day after the surgery I plowed through chapter 2 and was deep into chapter 3 when I paused to take a break. Junebug's nurse begged me to keep going.

"I'm into the story," she said. "I want to hear what happens next."

Exactly.

Whatever came next in the story, I wanted Juniper to long for more.

One morning we discovered that a new baby had arrived in 695, where the previous patient had vanished so ominously. The birth card identified the baby as a boy, but from where we sat, we couldn't make out his name. Even from a distance, though, we could see his intestines piled in a clear bag on top of his stomach.

His mother sat beside the incubator, alone in a wheelchair,

holding her gown closed in back with her hand. She was so young, maybe nineteen. Where was the little boy's father? Where were her parents? It made us ache to see her holding vigil all by herself. We wanted to talk to her, take her to the hospital cafeteria for a milk shake. But the invisible barriers restrained us.

That night, another baby was wheeled into 696. This incubator was closer, and I could read the card announcing that Baby Girl C. weighed 650 grams, slightly more than Juniper. I overheard the nurses saying that the baby's mother was still recovering from her C-section and that she spoke broken English. In the nurses' faces, I saw something that gave me pause—a flatness, as though they were trying to bury their thoughts.

Baby Girl C. had arrived from the operating room on a ventilator, but the next afternoon, the staff put her on a hi-fi vent, just like the one that was sending the rapid-fire puffs into Juniper's chest. As Kelley and I sat there, we could hear Baby Girl C.'s hi-fi machine rattling along with our daughter's.

Junebug was struggling through another bad day. The doctors had sedated her so she wouldn't dislodge the vent. Green stuff was draining from the tube in her belly, making it hard to balance her electrolytes. Her creatinine was up, which meant her kidneys were faltering, possibly because the doctors had her on four different antibiotics to fight the bacteria that had seeped into her torso through the hole in her bowels. The smallest infection, the doctors had warned us, could kill her. Now the team was debating how to ward off the bacteria without shutting down her kidneys.

Scott, our nurse that day, grimaced at the latest blood-gas report.

"Okay," he said, "so we're going to do a little baby makeover."

He repositioned the tape around her mouth, suctioned her endotracheal tube, straightened all the wires. He cupped her head in one hand and held her hand with the other, all the while watching the monitor. She gripped her ventilator tube with her right pinkie.

"Do you have any questions?" he asked.

Kelley looked at him.

"Would you agree she's the cutest baby you've ever worked on?"

"By far."

We were so focused on Junebug that we barely noticed when more nurses showed up to gather around Baby Girl C. in 696. A nurse practitioner hurried forward, and then several doctors. Then the mother arrived, still in her hospital gown, propped up by family members. Kelley and I tried not to stare, but the dread was so thick it crept toward us like a fog across water. Someone rolled a privacy screen in front of the incubator, and the nurses sent us out into the hall.

When we returned, the family was gone, and inside the incubator, underneath the blankets, was a shape, not moving. The blankets were expertly tucked and smoothed. On the floor were an empty alcohol packet and two crumpled tissues. The dead baby stayed there for hours. Scott and the other nurses did not speak of these things, did not look in the direction of the lump under the blanket, but their mouths grew tight.

I didn't want to imagine how many other babies had died in all of the incubators around us, or how many had died in the incubator where my daughter was sleeping now, or how many parents had sat exactly where we were sitting, holding a child gone cold and still.

Kelley

She had survived a week. Her nurse switched off the blue bilirubin lights and took the mask off her eyes. The black bruise under her left eye had faded into a dark crescent. Her eyelashes had grown longer. Her skin had lightened and thickened. She was no longer a glass shrimp, veiny and translucent.

We began to believe we could communicate with her. We spoke to her nonstop, and she never made a sound, though sometimes, by the contortions of her face, we could tell she was crying. Have you ever seen a terribly old man cry? The twisting, toothless, papery face, crumpling as though it could turn to dust.

A monitor charted her internal world and alarmed when something got out of whack, about every fifteen minutes. Tracy showed us how to read the screen's numbers and colors. The green line on top was her heart rate—sharp, even spikes like a picket fence. Her little heart ran faster than an adult's. Right now it was 145. The white number in the middle was her breathing, usually marked by an irregular squiggle. When it dipped low, it often meant she was asleep. Because today she was vibrating rather than breathing, that number was turned off.

The bottom number, charted in smooth aqua waves, measured the oxygen saturation in her blood. This number—they called it the sat number—was a critical and fascinating measure, because it provided an easy and constant assessment of her overall state.

If I saw nineties, Juniper earned an A. But anything below eighty-five was cause for intervention. Tracy would give her a second to recover, and if she didn't, she would turn the dial on the respirator to give her more oxygen. Giving more oxygen was dangerous because too much could make her blind. This was the first of dozens of cost-benefit analyses we would observe. Sometimes, a doctor would turn the oxygen up, and as soon as they left, Tracy would dial it back down.

It would be simplistic to say that this number reflected Juniper's mood, but that was how it seemed. If we touched her in a way she didn't like, by rubbing her skin, for example, the alarm would sound. If we cupped our hands around her head and feet, mimicking the boundaries and support of the womb, the number would rise.

We learned that very early babies have an almost animal ability to perceive the energy in a room. She lacked the development in her cerebral cortex to form an argument, but when she was bothered by something—a loud voice or a tense conversation—the oxygen level in her blood would drop, triggering her alarm. That's why the nurses had told us not to cry by the incubator.

One afternoon, when a nearby nurse complained about a participation grade she'd received in a college course, the sat number plummeted.

"She gave me a *six*. It's ten percent of the grade. She gave my friend who doesn't say anything an eight. I'm like *why*. And the girl who's Hispanic—and the teacher is Hispanic—got an eight."

Beep! Beep! Beep!

I shooed those nurses away, and I began to imagine what our interactions with each other would be like if we all walked around with a number like this on our foreheads, all fakery exposed.

> Tom: "It's a good thing you didn't see that movie. You would have hated it. So let me describe the alien abortion scene in agonizing detail for the next forty-five minutes, and then we can listen to a little *Jesus Christ Superstar.*"
> Me: Ding! Ding! Ding! Ding!

We became obsessed with the aqua number. Sometimes Tracy turned the monitor around so we couldn't see it.

The afternoon of Juniper's seventh day, Tom finished chapter 4, and Harry got his invitation to Hogwarts. I rested my head on his shoulder and stared at the saturation number. Juniper seemed pleased for Harry. The aqua number glowed ninety-seven...ninety-eight...But when Tom acted out the gruff voice of Hagrid the half giant, the alarms blared. Seventy-eight! Seventy-six! Seventy-four!!

I swatted Tom on the shoulder. "You're scaring the baby," I said. "Stop doing Hagrid."

"No way," Tom said. He kept reading.

Ding! Ding! Ding!

Juniper was listening. And, at a level beneath conscious thought, she was responding. Tom began to read every paragraph in a sweet, singsong voice. He vowed to coo even about Voldemort and the Dementors. The alarm stayed quiet.

Tom kept tapping on his iPad, drawing up his lists of the nurses' names, their responsibilities, and, I presumed, the names of their hamsters and cats. Within days, everyone knew who he was. He was the Good Dad. He was Father of the Year. Oh, and did you know he won a Pulitzer Prize? I could slip in and out of the NICU unnoticed, just another dazed, short-tempered, hormonal mom. All my flaws and insecurities were on display. I wore my pajamas every day. I didn't have the energy to try to impress anyone.

Mom is stressed, someone noted in the chart.

One morning I watched Tracy dab K-Y Jelly on Juniper's forehead to attach a tiny bow. I didn't know what to make of all the pumps and machines, and I strained to follow a lot of the medical babble, but I understood the meaning in that small gesture.

This is your daughter. Get to know her.

I used medical tape to stick a photo of Tom and me to her incubator, so when her eyes opened, she would know who her parents were, and so the doctors and nurses who interacted with her would know she was loved. I thought they might subconsciously fight harder for a girl who had a future and a home and a family. I scoured the Internet for the softest possible blankets. I got her a tiny iPod and loaded it with womb sounds, to fill in the spaces when we couldn't be there. What more could I do to connect with a little girl who couldn't see or eat or scream? How do you parent a baby in a plastic box?

Juniper survived a second week. On Tuesday, her fourteenth day, Tom's sister Susi was flying in from Indiana, and his brother Ben was coming in from New York. I dragged myself out of bed so I could be at the hospital early. At rounds, we learned that she now weighed 650 grams—1 pound 7 ounces. It was hard to say how much of the 3 ounces she'd gained was real and how much was just extra fluid.

"We are not getting adequate calories into her," one of the doctors said.

A nutritionist explained the balancing act: her belly had a hole in it, so they gave her liquid nutrition through a vein, but they could only put in so much fluid without throwing her body off kilter, and they could only make the solution so concentrated. She needed protein, but too much could stress her kidneys. She needed fat, but too much could exacerbate her lung disease.

Diane explained that every system in her body—brain, lungs, kidney, belly, heart—was running its own marathon, and the doctors were trying to get all of them to the finish line together. But those systems all interacted with one another in complicated ways. Every treatment exacted a cost. If any one of them failed, the baby would die.

I silently thanked my high school chemistry teacher, Mr. James Ford. He had warned us the day would come when those dreary textbook chapters would come alive, crashing into our lives with terrible relevance. *"It's chemistry, people!"* he'd shout, trying to make us see that the things we take for granted, like fire and breath, are chemical reactions, collisions of elements. Now I saw him, his kind grin and bushy mustache aquiver with excitement. My education in the sciences was fundamental at best, but I more or less understood the doctors' metric patter. And more, I understood what Mr. Ford had been trying to tell me, that science and life are inseparable. That the chemicals dripping through the IV tubes and the love I felt watching it happen were somehow connected, somewhere I couldn't see.

Juniper's lungs looked cloudy on the X-ray. That usually meant the lung was collapsing or scarred. But her blood tests showed that she was taking in oxygen, that she was neither too acidic nor too basic, that somehow her body's internal combustion engine was sputtering along. She had come off the noisy vibrating ventilator. The doctors gradually reduced her oxygen to a reasonable level. She looked better than the X-ray would indicate.

"Let's follow the baby, not the X-ray," Dr. Shakeel said.

There existed here a tension between the machines and the interpreters reading the reports. Dr. Shakeel articulated it so clearly.

"Follow the baby," she had said. The baby who couldn't speak, leading them all along, showing them the way. They turned their dials. They tested her blood. They read the numbers.

"Phenomenal," Dr. Shakeel said.

They charted five poops. "Excellent," Dr. Shakeel said.

I reached in and put my hand over Juniper's bare back, and I could feel the air moving in her lungs. A respiratory therapist came by to check the ventilator settings.

"For as little as she is, she's doing great," she said.

I headed to the awful pumping closet, with its single mini-fridge. I still wasn't making much milk—maybe an ounce here and there. It still took hours. My body must have been confused. Where had the baby gone? Why wasn't she nursing? What was this groaning plastic contraption?

You're pathetic.

You're pathetic.

You're nobody's mom.

In the pod, parenthood was cold and mechanical. I understood why some parents fled. My hormones were raging. I had so many stabilizing forces in my life that allowed me to hang on. If any one of them had been broken or missing, I could not imagine how I would have coped: if I didn't have Tom, if I lived far away, if I couldn't miss work, if I had to take the bus, if I had other kids. If I had not wanted this baby so badly, and loved her so damn much.

I was starting to see how nurses like Tracy and doctors like Dr. Shakeel found ways to seize the tiniest wisps of humanity and breathe into them until they sparked.

Tom called my cell phone. When I picked up, I knew he could hear the awful pump groaning on and on in the background. Gross.

"They want you to hold her today," he said.

I didn't understand.

Hold who?

I hadn't been expecting this for at least a few more weeks, when she came off the ventilator. Our nurse said that it was Tuesday, the day they change the incubators so they can be cleaned. They had to move the baby anyway; why not hold her while she was out? So within a few hours, I was settling into the blue vinyl recliner and watching as a physical therapist spent half an hour massaging and calming our baby to prepare her for the journey back to my body. The distance was maybe three feet. It felt so much greater than that.

The therapist's name was Ana Maria Jara, and she explained what should have been obvious. Babies need their moms. Doctors knew that even the most vulnerable held their body temperature better, breathed better, digested food better, and generally fared better if they spent time skin to skin with their parents. It was still a controversial idea for the tiniest babies. Some nurses, Tracy included, worried that the touchy-feely impulses could overshadow basic concerns, like protecting the airway and preventing infection. In the early days of neonatology, parents never got to hold their babies. But now, All Children's had twenty-four-hour visitation and people like Ana Maria.

We watched her slowly and quietly massage Juniper with the tip of her finger. Juniper's face contorted into a silent cry, then relaxed. She melted into Ana Maria's hands.

"They don't listen to your words," Ana Maria explained. "They listen to your feelings." She was a Preemie Whisperer.

She spoke softly to Juniper in English and in Spanish.

"Qué pasa, niña?"

She gathered all the tubes and wires so nothing would tug at the baby when she was moved. Tom recorded it all on his iPhone. I just grinned, crazily.

"You are going to go on a little trip," Ana Maria told Juniper.

When all was ready, the therapist lifted the baby and moved her slowly, on a straight plane, being careful not to jostle the ventilator tube even a few millimeters. Finally she placed her on my chest and tucked her inside my shirt. Her feet pressed into my ribs, and her head rested right under my chin. I put my hand on her back. Ana Maria told me to press just a little, because babies love to feel secure. On the monitor, I saw that Juniper began to breathe easier and easier. Ninety-seven... ninety-eight... ninety-nine.

It really did feel like I was whole again. I could forget the wires, the monitors, the tubes and bandages, the alarms, the other babies, the swirl of science and of statistics and probability and loss. I was holding my baby girl. She was wearing a pink hat. Her hands were curled under her chin. She seemed content. She could feel my heart. She was warm under my hand. She was the same little girl who had squirmed inside my body. The one

I'd pleaded with on the bathroom floor. The one who had been ripped away.

We needed each other. Here was a thing I could do.

Just as she was settled, Tom's brother and sister arrived from the airport. Everyone gathered around, taking in how tiny the baby was, how wrinkled and dark, and how safe she looked. I don't know if she felt it, but she was part of a family then. Susi and Ben greeted her not as a mishap or as a possibility, but wholeheartedly, as one of a tribe.

Ana Maria told me to breathe deeply and calmly and the baby would copy me and we would fall into a rhythm together. I tried to project strength and comfort with every breath. I didn't know if Juniper picked up on all that, or if she even knew where she was. But I wanted to believe she did.

She was so bony and so light. Like a baby bird, I thought. I breathed for both of us.

Later, someone told me the truth. There had been no urgent need to clean the incubator. Ana Maria and our nurse had spoken to Dr. Shakeel that morning and made a case. They all agreed that Juniper was having a rare good day.

And every mom should get to hold her baby at least once while she is still alive.

Tom

The honeymoon was such a distant memory that it no longer seemed real. Juniper's bad days outnumbered her good ones. I would be working to understand one complication when two more setbacks would be announced at morning rounds. The doctors were still having trouble maintaining her blood pressure. Her bone marrow was not yet capable of producing enough red blood cells, so she was becoming anemic. She needed transfusions every few days.

One of her umbilical lines had been removed after it stopped working due to the size of her veins. The other umbilical line was failing, too. The team needed a central line that they could rely on, so they had inserted a catheter called a PICC into one of her arms. Every time another line or another needle went into her body, the risk of infection grew. The floor beneath our feet, the handles on the doors, the buttons on the elevator—every surface was swimming in germs that could kill her. All it would take was for one of us to step away for a minute and then forget to thoroughly scrub our hands again when we came back.

Tracy was almost psychic. One of her priorities was figuring out which of the IVs or other lines running into Junebug's body was going to give out next. She would start planning how to get another line up and running before the current one became useless. If they couldn't get meds inside the baby, the situation could turn catastrophic. When Tracy needed to put in a new IV, she asked us to step into the hall.

"I get nervous with you guys watching me," she said.

We had believed that Tracy was unshakable. If inserting a new line gave her the jitters, it obviously wasn't simple at all. I tried to see the task through Tracy's eyes: the filament of Junebug's vein, the catheter a thread of silk. The meds pulsing through that IV, headed for Junebug's heart, the heart pumping the meds into the rest of her body. The flow suddenly halting when the catheter broke through the vein, sending the meds pouring into parts of her body where they weren't meant to go.

Junebug was one of the smallest and most underdeveloped babies in the hospital. It was not an exaggeration to say that at that moment, she remained one of the smallest human beings in the world.

To Kelley and me, she had begun to look almost normal, even when we sanitized our wedding rings and slipped them over her foot and ankle. Whenever we saw full-term babies, we were stunned at their gargantuan proportions. One morning I looked up from my chair at Junebug's incubator and saw one of these giants being wheeled in. I made a pretense of heading for the bathroom to get a closer look.

The mystery boy was pink and chubby. His ID card declared his weight to be 4.11 kilograms, almost seven times the size of Junebug. I pictured him stomping through the streets of Tokyo, towering over buildings, crushing buses under his big baby feet. I texted Kelley, who was at home pumping milk.

4.11 kg is a nine-pound baby.

Fat ass, she replied.

What kinda self-respecting NICU admits a nine-pound baby?

He's a fraud.

I couldn't remember the last time we had laughed.

Kelley and I had fallen into a routine. Not a healthy one, but a routine just the same. At dawn I would go into All Children's to be there for the hands-on sessions and for morning rounds. Kelley hated being left behind, strapped to the pump. Some mornings when I returned to the house she could barely speak, glaring at me with teary eyes.

On Easter morning, I went into the NICU early as usual. Volunteers had made Easter baskets for all the babies on the floor. I put ours aside so Kelley could open it when she came in. Tracy, back on duty, was wearing purple scrubs with a zebra-print shirt underneath and her zebra-striped clogs. She encouraged me to change Junebug's diaper. I had changed thousands of Nat's and Sam's diapers, but I had no experience with girls. The smallest diapers the NICU had were too big for my daughter, so Tracy taught me how to fold the top and make it snug and then slowly negotiate my way under the wires. Then she handed me some wipes.

"Front to back. That's all you need to know."

I wondered how many clueless fathers she'd tutored. I discovered that Juniper had no butt to speak of, just a single wrinkle stretching lengthwise along each cheek. I fumbled with the diaper tabs, fastening them too tight. When I tried to fix them, one of the tabs tore away.

"Takes practice," Tracy said. "You'll get there."

Later that morning I went home and gave Kelley an Easter

card and some chocolates. She barely smiled. We got back to the NICU just before noon. Kelley pulled back the quilt on the top of Junebug's incubator and knew instantly that something was wrong.

"How did my baby grow another chin?"

For a second I thought she was kidding. Then I saw that Junebug's chest and neck were swollen.

"Why didn't someone notice?" she said.

I knew she didn't mean Tracy, because we both had absolute confidence in Tracy. I felt my face go red.

Tracy explained that Junebug's PICC line had become dislodged from her vein and had been pumping lipids and nutrients into her upper chest. She said she'd been lucky to catch it so quickly. She'd taken out the PICC—the team would have to replace it. Tracy had been hurrying over to tell us about the infiltration, but Kelley had spotted it before she'd had the chance.

Kelley caught things that I missed, no question. If Junebug's stomach was slightly splotchy, her mother saw it before I did. If the baby was restless, Kelley moved to comfort her before the monitor sounded. Though Kelley never said it directly, my powers of observation were inferior—humiliating, if you're a reporter allegedly trained in the divinity of small details. At the same time, it irritated Kelley that my early mornings with Junebug had made me more experienced with certain tasks. Kelley was the mother, not me, and she did not appreciate having to play catch-up. That night, when I coached her on how to change the baby's diaper, repeating what Tracy had told me, Kelley fixed me with an evil eye. When I reminded her to sanitize her hands before lifting the baby, she seethed.

When we landed in the NICU, I had hoped the two of us would comfort each other through this crisis. But my narrative of solidarity was already in tatters. We weren't helping each other ride the riptide of emotions. We were dragging each other under.

My patience was almost gone. Beneath my exhaustion, I harbored a secret anger. I was brooding about the day Kelley rode the bike with Muppet loping alongside. I had begged her not to do it, and she had ignored me. She had always mocked my cautious tendencies, as if I were a doddering old man. I fought to keep my spiteful thoughts in check. If I let them pour out, especially when both of us were so vulnerable, they would burn through our marriage.

We still had our pact, Kelley and I. Only one of us could lose it at any given moment. But so far my wife was monopolizing the available freak-out time. I couldn't understand why she kept giving in to despair, day after day, while she expected me to hold her up. I was faithfully going to the NICU early every morning. I was the one writing down what the doctors said and asking them the questions she wanted answered. I was learning how to take care of the baby, reading to the baby, singing to her and talking to her at all hours. And yet Kelley resented me.

Late one night, as we were going to bed, I snapped.

"Why do you keep bitching and moaning? On and on and on. Does it help? Does it really make you feel better?"

As soon as the words left my mouth, I wanted to yank them back.

Kelley

I stayed up late, raging in my head, and also hating myself because I was mad about—what, exactly? Losing to him in the Parent Olympics?

Tom was spackling over his grief and terror. Baking all those cookies, passing around the recipe, as if the person our daughter needed in her life was Betty Crocker.

I drifted off into a nightmare. I saw myself in our bathroom. The baby had just been cut out of me, and I was still trying to deliver the afterbirth. I was writhing in my own blood, and Tom told me I was boring. I went to the hospital to see Juniper, but the guards wouldn't let me in.

The next day, both of us calmer, I tried to explain the emotional quicksand that tugged me when Tom left for the hospital in the mornings. The gratitude and relief that he was on duty. The disgust with myself for staying behind, strapped to that tormenting machine. I was wasting all those hours, missing her short life, probably for nothing. What if those hours were all I had?

Part of me, the part bogged in the deepest self-loathing, wondered if the machine was the real enemy. Was I just too weak to face the NICU, the monitors, the nurses, and even my own struggling daughter? Was I such a failure of a mother that I would leave her there alone?

Tom sat on the edge of the bed, which smelled like sour milk. His face softened, and I knew he wasn't mad anymore.

"I could not do this without you," he said.

You're the one who willed this baby into being, he told me. You carried her in your body for five months, but you carried her inside of you for years. You believed in her and you fought for her. You kicked my ass all the way to the altar, knocking me past my fears of being too old. You listened to all my complaining about the Room of Requirement and endured God knows how many people messing inside you with catheters and cameras, and you seduced another woman into giving us her eggs, all because you had a vision of this baby in your arms.

I was crying now, smearing tears and snot all over his T-shirt.

"Junebug," he said, "is here only because of you. If you're not the most ferocious mother on the planet, you tell me who is."

I saw a counselor. I needed to vent and rage at someone, and I knew it should not be Tom. I spewed and cried for the entire hour, paid the ninety dollars, and left feeling guilty for transferring such raw horror onto another human being.

I knew Tom was right. Hormones were screwing with me. I was a mess, but I was the only mother Juniper had.

"Come on," Tom said one morning soon after. "Get your ass out of bed."

Tom

The tunnel led us away from the surface of the earth, away from what we had thought were our lives. We would wind downward farther and farther, telling ourselves that surely we were nearing the bottom, and then we would see the path stretching before us, twisting into the distance, carrying us toward something we knew we could not bear.

We slept without sleeping, falling and falling. I drifted off behind the wheel at stoplights, standing in the kitchen, in whatever chair I landed. Stepping onto the hospital's elevators, I had grown to despise the recorded voices of the children so eager to remind us what direction we were headed.

"Going down!" one would chirp.

"Going down, yes!" I would say out loud. "Down to the ninth circle of hell."

My only refuge now came in the hours when I read to my daughter. We were speeding through the middle chapters of *The Sorcerer's Stone*. Harry had survived his first lesson on the broomstick and his first Quidditch match, and Junebug and I soared with him above the ramparts and the towers, grasping for the Golden Snitch. The further we ventured into the book, the more she seemed to enjoy it. When I read, her sat number consistently stayed in the upper nineties. When I stopped, the number often dropped.

"You'd better keep going," one of the nurses told me. "She's into it."

While I lost myself in the halls of Hogwarts, Kelley kept her focus on the baby. She muttered and stewed through an entire weekend, insisting Junebug's belly looked swollen again. I couldn't see it. Tracy, Diane, Dr. Shakeel—all the people we trusted most—were off duty. Kelley asked a nurse practitioner to take a look, but the woman had seemed distracted and barely glanced at the baby. The next morning, when Diane was back, I sought her out to ask what we should do if we felt someone on the staff was not listening. I pushed away my tendency to be diplomatic and channeled some of Kelley's directness.

"We're not afraid of being a pain in the ass," I told Diane. "But we can't tell when being a pain in the ass is useful."

Diane laughed.

"You should be a pain in the ass if you see something alarming."

That afternoon, the doctors discovered that Junebug's intestines had perforated again, and a surgeon inserted two more drains into her abdomen. Kelley had been right. For several days she had known something was wrong. I hadn't caught it, but neither had anyone else.

I read only a little to Junebug that afternoon. The second surgery had worn her out, and she needed to rest. The nurses were no longer commenting on her feistiness. All the fight seemed to have been squeezed out of her. The team could not maintain her blood pressure, and even when they turned up her oxygen to 90 percent, barely any of it was reaching her lungs.

That evening, Kelley and I slipped out for dinner and then hurried back to All Children's to be there for the start of the night shift. We were just coming off the interstate, with the hospital looming beside the highway, the lights on the sixth floor waiting, when a crushing thought occurred to me. What if Juniper died before I had a chance to read her the last chapter? What if she never got to hear what happened to Harry and Ron and Hermione? Suddenly all the fear and sorrow I'd been trying to keep at bay came roaring up through my chest and into my throat. I couldn't breathe. I couldn't stop my shoulders from heaving. I pulled over and collapsed against the steering wheel.

"What's wrong, baby?" said Kelley, reaching over to rub my shoulder. "Tell me what it is."

I could not say it out loud.

Sam, still fighting bronchitis, had not yet met Junebug. If she died now, she would never know her brother, and he would never feel her samurai grip on his finger. Mother's Day would be here soon, and we would spend it at our daughter's grave. Junebug would never meet Muppet or hug her neck. She would never see her room at home that Kelley had made so beautiful with the orange monkey rug and the shelves bursting with picture books. Halloween would come, and she wouldn't get to dress as a ladybug or go trick-or-treating. At Christmas, she would not see the lights on the tree. Every year, we hung ornaments with childhood photos of Nat and Sam and a picture of Kelley in the snow as a little girl, another of me as a baby squirming on Santa's lap. What photo would we frame of Junebug? Without her, would we even have the heart to put up a tree? She would never grow older. She would never know anything but the darkness of the box she was living in now and the darkness of the box that came next.

It was the unfinished book that struck me as the most unfair. If Junebug died without us finishing the last chapter of *The Sor-*

cerer's Stone, she would never know what a happy ending felt like. She would be trapped in a wasteland of no resolution.

As we arrived in the NICU and walked to her incubator, I was overcome again and ran out to the hall. Through the windows I watched the sun go down, the blur of headlights and taillights hurtling toward other worlds. Now I understood why Kelley had found it so difficult these past weeks to enter this place. She had been facing the truth, and I had been hiding from it. Somehow I had convinced myself that I was being brave, but I'd only been playing a more subtle version of make-believe.

It was dark outside. My reflection stared back at me from the black windows. I could not believe how ancient I looked, how ridiculous with my puffy eyes and silver hair, uncombed for days. I told myself that I was useless. A fool who believed he could protect his daughter by reading her a book.

When I went back in, Kelley asked if I wanted to hold Junebug's hand. I told myself that my daughter needed me to be strong and that I could not be crying when my fingers touched hers, or else she would know. I took a deep breath and reached inside the incubator. Junebug was out of it, somewhere far away from us now, dreaming whatever she dreamed.

"We need you to come home," I said. "Come home. Come home."

At last, I opened *The Sorcerer's Stone* where we'd left off, at the top of page 200, where Harry and Ron open their Christmas presents and Harry unwraps the invisibility cloak that had once belonged to his father. I read quietly, taking the sentences inside me and then letting them out, breathing along with every beat and every pause.

It was the only thing I knew to do.

Kelley

I couldn't stop thinking about the dead baby in 696—the one who had died across the aisle, and then lain so still under the sheet. I thought about those parents, stumbling out of the pod, into a life that must have felt as though it had no bottom. I would imagine when that day would come for me.

I saw it so clearly. The nurses would sit me down in the blue vinyl recliner. They would turn to Juniper and gently unpeel the tape from her face. They would unhook the wires, one by one. They'd pull the tubes out of her mouth, and out of her nose. They would shut off the monitor, and the screen would go dark. They would gently lift my daughter out of the incubator, wrap her in a blanket, and lay her in my arms. She would weigh nothing. She'd be sedated, so she wouldn't struggle, but she'd gasp. Tom would want to hold her, but I would cling to her as long as I could. I would be a mother for a moment. I would try to say something a dying baby would need her mother to say. "You are not alone. I love you more than the world." I would memorize her face. I would be terrified of forgetting. We would pass her back and forth until she grew cold and mottled and gray. It would take longer than you'd think. The stethoscope would leave an imprint on her chest.

We would walk away not knowing who we were.

Tom

Watching the baby that night was like witnessing a plane crashing over and over. The aqua number on her monitor kept dropping. Her blood pressure was dangerously low, a possible sign of infection. Dr. Eeyore was on duty, and he and the nurse and a respiratory tech worked on her for hours. They repositioned her vent tube, working it deeper to increase the airflow, and ordered more antibiotics, and did everything they could to raise her sat number. She finally stabilized at around nine-thirty, and Kelley and I went home to get some sleep. We knew that the next day could very well be our daughter's last, and we would need whatever strength we had left.

Once I lay down, I collapsed into a dream unlike any I'd ever had. I was a contestant on a TV game show, standing next to Junebug's incubator on a bright stage trimmed in blue neon and flashing with lights that reminded me of *Who Wants to Be a Millionaire?* Though the host never said it out loud, the prize of the show was clearly my daughter's survival. I was to play multiple rounds, and if I kept winning, she had a chance to live. If I lost a round, she died.

The dream went on forever. Music blared through studio speakers. The audience roared and applauded through round after round as the cameras zoomed in on Junebug's sleeping face and on her monitor, showing her vital signs for everyone at home to see and speculate about. I wanted to complain that she needed quiet, that all this noise wasn't good for her, but there was never a chance to get in a word with all the cheering and the canned music and the scripted banter from the host. I couldn't hear if the alarms were going off, and I had to focus so intently on the game that I had no chance to study her monitor. Both of us were drowning in the show's artificial elation.

Kelley was not onstage with me, and the lights were so blinding I could not find her face in the audience. But during one round, Nat and Sam were called up and asked to stand on either side of the incubator, and my task was to somehow connect my boys with their little sister through rays of light, forming spokes in a glowing wheel. When I completed that challenge, the audience erupted with applause, and suddenly I was in another round that required me to identify cities around the world where Junebug might live as an adult if she survived the game.

I was still inside the show when I heard a buzzing. It was Kelley's cell phone, vibrating on the shelf behind our bed. I looked at the screen.

All Children's Hospital.

2:17 a.m.

I answered, and Dr. Eeyore apologized for waking me. I felt bad for identifying him that way in my head, this man toiling in the middle of the night to save our daughter. Kelley leaned in to listen along, and through the phone we could hear Dr. Germain measuring his words even more carefully than usual. They were having trouble with Juniper's breathing again, he said, and had put her back on the hi-fi ventilator. They had turned up the oxygen to 100 percent, but it wasn't enough. They couldn't maintain her blood pressure. They were having trouble with her urine output. All the signs pointed toward a massive infection.

"How close do you live to the hospital?" he asked.

"Oh God," said Kelley.

I was still groggy. Being lurched out of the game-show dream and thrown into this conversation was making it hard for me to really hear what Dr. Germain was telling me. Knowing that the high oxygen rate could blind Junebug, I asked him how long they could keep her at 100 percent before they had to worry about damaging her eyes.

"Immediately," he said. "Her retinal development is a long-term issue. I'm focused on the short term right now."

This time I heard it. Juniper was dying. Dr. Germain just didn't want to use the word. His first priority, the doctor said, was to make sure she made it through the night. He sounded depleted. Before Junebug was born, he had warned us of the odds and the dangers, had quoted us percentages of risk. Now he was doing his best to help our daughter beat the odds.

"She's a very, very sick little girl. I'm very concerned about her right now."

Before hanging up, Dr. Germain assured us he would call if there was any change. Once again, he asked how far away we lived.

We arrived back at the hospital just after 3:30 a.m., the fear written so plain on our faces that the people we passed looked away. In the elevator, another one of those disembodied, demonic children taunted us.

"Going up! Sixth floor!"

When we peered into Junebug's incubator, she was sleeping

hard, her arms and legs splayed wide like she'd been knocked out in a prizefight. Holly, her night nurse, told us it was best to let her rest, because the team had been working on her for so long and had just managed to stabilize her. But her oxygen was still up high, near 100 percent, and Holly was worried about the damage. It was as though we were watching her go blind right there.

"My little Junebug," Kelley said. "Her poor little eyeballs."

Holly had another piece of bad news. Trying to counter the acidity of Junebug's blood gases, the doctors had prescribed sodium bicarbonate to be pumped through an IV. But that night, the IV had burst through the vein and leaked the bicarb into the flesh of her right hand.

The nurse had caught the infiltration quickly, but by then the bicarb had eaten away a sizable chunk of tissue, perhaps the size of a dime—huge, on such a tiny hand. If Junebug survived, we would eventually need to take her to the hospital's plastic surgeon, the one who played the piano in the hospital lobby, to repair the damage.

Holly said she'd never had a patient suffer an infiltration like it.

"In sixteen years, that's a first for me," she told us. "That bicarb is nasty stuff."

Normally the NICU did not encourage parents to spend the night. But tonight was different. I rolled over an easy chair for Kelley, and she dropped into it and began to cry. I found a blanket to drape over her. I sat down beside her and stared into the darkness of our daughter's box and listened to the frantic hum of her hi-fi vent. Alarms echoed through the unit, as though every baby in the world were struggling. I couldn't help noticing that when other nurses walked by—nurses who had taken care of Junebug and obviously cared about her—they would not glance in our direction.

Their faces were tight, with that flatness I had come to know all too well.

Kelley

Dr. Shakeel took over that morning. She told us that surgery might be the last option. Whatever was going on in Juniper's belly wasn't healing, and either infection or pressure or some other fallout was shutting down the rest of her body, too. Dr. Shakeel had talked to the surgeon, who had insisted she did not want to operate on a baby so small. The operation would be more complex than putting in drains. The surgeon, Dr. Beth Walford, would have to cut her open and look for areas of dead or burst bowel; then she would have to remove those and do her best to put all the pieces back together.

Dr. Walford told us that she almost never performed major surgery on such a tiny baby. The doctors would have to stabilize her enough to get her on a regular ventilator, because they couldn't operate on a baby who was vibrating. The surgery would require a trip to the operating room, and that trip alone could kill her. And once the team cut her open, her skin was so delicate that Dr. Walford might not be able to sew her shut. The doctor wanted to make sure we understood.

"How many babies this size have you performed this surgery on?" I asked.

Dr. Walford was brave enough to look us in the eye.

"Two who were under a kilo," she said.

Juniper was still barely half that weight.

"And of those two, how many survived?"

She paused.

"One."

Dr. Shakeel had been weighing the options all morning. She knew the surgery was a huge risk and a last resort. It would almost certainly kill our daughter. But what other option was there? Juniper was dying anyway. She asked us what we wanted to do.

We couldn't know. Again, we were desperate for guidance. We had to leave it in the doctor's hands. The answers were not in the textbook or in the research.

Later, Dr. Shakeel told me that she had debated it in her head for an hour. *I've adjusted the vent. I've bumped up the drips. What else can I do?*

Impossible decisions were part of the job. She learned all she could, made the best decision she could, and then never second-guessed herself. Her faith told her that God was in control. She let him guide her.

She knew numbers never told the whole story. "Follow the baby," she always said. So that morning, torn about what to do, she went to Bed 692 and peered inside.

Juniper's eyes were just starting to open, after being fused since birth. Now she opened them, wide, and looked right at the doctor.

Dr. Shakeel saw a baby who was almost a month old and not yet two pounds, whose body was shutting down, who was sedated and groggy and in so much pain, but was fighting to engage with the world. Her eyes were opening and closing.

Opening and closing. Dr. Shakeel felt her saying, *I'm here. I'm here.*

Juniper French was declaring herself.

Dr. Shakeel got the surgeon on the phone.

We called Mike and Roy. Tom wanted Juniper baptized, which startled me. We had never even been to church together. In no time, Roy was there in his Rays cap, holding a cup of sterile hospital water. He said baptisms signified beginnings, not endings, and sprinkled Juniper's forehead. Mike signed a certificate from Roy's Catholic church as a witness. We wanted to ask Mike to be Juniper's godfather, but given our confused spirituality, we weren't even sure what the title meant. Whatever it was, he was already playing the part.

Soon our baby was headed to the operating room. The nurses were busying about, connecting the mobile ventilator and the portable monitor. I held her hand. She was looking at me. Right *at* me, in a way she never had before. Her eyes were dark pools, taking in everything. Taking in my face, and my voice.

"It won't always be like this, baby.

"There are some things you need to know about. Like ice cream. You won't believe the chocolate milk shake at Coney Island Grill. And at home, there's a goofy dog named Muppet who will lick you too much, and her breath stinks but you can tell her all your secrets and she'll never share. You have your own room, with a zebra on the wall and a round crib and a soft rocking chair where I will hold you. We'll take you to a Springsteen concert, if he can keep going long enough, and you can hear 'Waitin' On a Sunny Day' and watch him slide across the stage. We'll take you to Fort De Soto and you can mush your toes in the sand. Someday you'll ride a horse bareback in the sun, and you'll go so fast your eyes will water. You'll dance in your jammies. You'll hold my hand and I'll take you to school, and when the bell rings at the end of the day, I'll be waiting for you."

They wheeled her in her incubator as far as the operating room, and we walked alongside. Finally we could follow her no farther. We stopped so we could say good-bye.

"You can give her a kiss," Tracy said.

Until now I had not tortured myself with the thought that I might never kiss my daughter. I knew the odds were good that when I saw her again, she would be cold.

I leaned in, and kissed her tiny little forehead, and lingered there, trying to communicate everything I couldn't say, to be near her, to hold on to her, to breathe her in.

Tom gave her a kiss, and they wheeled her away.

We walked the halls. They'd given us one of those pagers like you get at the Cheesecake Factory and told us the surgery would take a couple of hours. My mind played a game as I walked. I saw cute kids in the elevator or the cafeteria, and I tried to guess what was wrong with them. I wondered if, whatever it was, I would trade my problems for theirs. Big-eyed blond kid in the elevator? Blood disease. Cute freckled kid in the parking garage? Heart trouble. Baby in the stroller in a full-body cast? Brittle bones.

I knew I would not trade. Even if she died, trying to save her had been the right decision. We'd gotten to know her. We'd let her hear our voices, and hear music, and feel our hands on her. Some of the greatest moments of my life had been tucked inside this misery. Memorizing her face. Holding her hand. Feeling her warm and weightless form on my chest. Reading her a story. Writing "Mom" on a consent form. Every act, no matter how mundane, affirmed that this child belonged to me, that I belonged to her. If those moments were not so precious, there would be no terror, no cruelty, in seeing them snatched away.

"She's my daughter," Tom said. "I wouldn't change any of it."

There are worse things than watching your baby die like this, I told myself.

Forgetting your child in the backseat of a car on a hot day, and finding her when it was too late. That would be worse. But that happens to good people, all the time. Pulling a dead two-year-old out of a swimming pool would be worse. Losing a child at any age greater than hers would be worse, because every day makes letting go so much harder. But these things were happening to people right now, in this building. They happened here every day. They had been happening long before I had reason to pay attention.

Every day, thousands of prayers were launched into the universe, to God, to Jehovah, and to Señor Jesucristo y mi Virgen María Guadalupe. Love and faith and grief were part of this place. In the hospital chapel, the prayer book told the story.

I am really scared. All I do is pray.
She doesn't know it, but she is my world.
Well, God. I've been praying every day, but sometimes
    the answer is not what we want. I trust you. Take
    care of her.
Thank you, Lord, for one more day.

I thought about all the people who'd told us they were praying for our baby. Churches we'd never set foot in. Some of Tom's friends had gotten word to a mosque in India, where seven hundred people gathered just to pray for Juniper. Some spiritual types in Atlanta were meditating on it. My friend Lucia set up an altar on her fireplace mantel, with candles burning. The people at Preacher's Barbecue held hands and prayed for Juniper before they handed us our ribs. I began to think of all this prayer as a big cloud rising over all of us, sheltering us.

I didn't know it yet, but somewhere in that cloud was the voice of Dr. Shakeel.

The afternoon of the surgery, in a small room near the NICU, Dr. Shakeel kneeled on her prayer rug and prayed for our baby. She had exhausted her expertise, pushed technology to its limit. Now she surrendered.

She faced east, toward Mecca. She spoke to the one who creates life and brings death, the one with the power to heal. She told God he was in control. She asked for his help. She touched her forehead to the ground.

PART FOUR

Dark Star

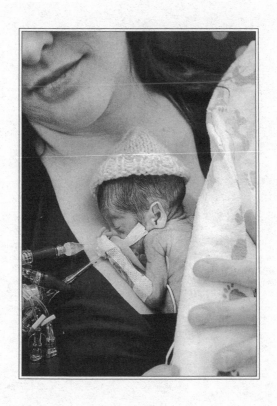

Tom

I tried not to think, not to wonder, not to hope, not to predict, not to imagine. I had never had a chance to truly hold my daughter, to feel her face against my shoulder and inhale the scent of her and know the reality of her sleeping in my arms. I did not want to contemplate the likelihood that I would get to hold her that very afternoon, just once, before they put her in the ground.

During the surgery Kelley and her mother and I waited downstairs in the hospital cafeteria, waited for the red lights to flash on the Cheesecake Factory buzzer, waited on and on. Kelley kept saying she wanted to throw up, and her mother kept sighing, and I tried to avoid the clock on the wall. I had never hated time as much as I did that day. I wanted it to fast-forward to the moment when we heard the news. I wanted it to slow down, so that we would have longer to believe she might still be alive.

I had spent my life studying stories and their endings. As a kid, I used to sit up with my dad and watch movies and guess how it was all going to turn out. Would the police catch the psycho killer? Would the hero survive the train plunging into the ravine? Even then, I was good at guessing which way the sequence would turn. Now I was living inside a story I could neither control nor predict.

The red lights on the buzzer flashed. We went to a conference room upstairs and waited. That was the worst, those final few minutes.

The door opened, and as Dr. Walford entered, I read her face and saw a weariness that made my stomach drop. Our daughter was alive, she told us, but the news was not good. The surgeon explained that when she had opened Junebug's abdomen, her intestines had been so inflamed and matted that it had been useless to attempt any repair.

"When I touched them, they fell apart."

Kelley and I struggled to speak. We asked if there was any hope. Was it possible the problem could be fixed after she grew bigger and stronger?

"For the moment," Dr. Walford said, "all we can do is wait and see how she does."

We were grateful for even another hour with our daughter. We went upstairs to the NICU and watched her sleep. On my phone I began to compose an e-mail update for Nat and Sam and Roy and Mike and my family. I was so exhausted that I kept falling asleep in midsentence, lapsing into gibberish.

they put in a couple new drains in hopes that will clear it up. This seems a little unlikely to
Usf
l

As I nodded off, my thumb accidentally hit "send." A few seconds later I woke up and tried again.

But Junebug's blood pressure is up, and she's peeing agai
One more time.
Thanks for the love and support, every
I fell asleep in the chair.

Kelley

The next morning Tom and I arrived at the hospital and made the familiar walk across the covered corridor from the parking garage. The hospital gleamed with a surreal cleanliness and optimism. The halls were lined with cartoonish sculptures of pelicans and dolphins. As always, children sat astride them, while moms tugged them toward the lab for blood work or to the registration desk for tonsillectomies. The art along the walls was designed for kids. Now the cheerfulness felt forced and mocking. We passed the strange, three-dimensional sheepdog who wore sunglasses and hung his head out a car window. Something about that dog creeped me out. We passed the colorful metal fish, swimming along the wall toward the elevator. I wondered if, by the time we left that night, I'd no longer be a mom.

I could barely remember the things I had done before, or what I had loved. I loved Tom, more than ever now that we were aligned in a common battle. I loved the people who had stood with us beside the plastic box. I loved Mike and Jennifer and Ben and Roy. But I didn't care about work, which had once defined and guided me. I didn't care about food, or breath, or sex, or the dog, or money, or myself. The baby, this hint of a girl, shut out all the rest. I had never heard her voice or seen her smile, but I knew her better than I knew my own terrible, conflicted heart.

The security guard glanced at our badges. BED 692. 4/12/11. JUNIPER FRENCH. NICU. Short-timers got stickers, good for a day. Our badges meant our child was not leaving. We belonged in a place we wanted to flee.

We were waved through the locked double doors into Six South; past the sign-in desk, where I wrote "Mom" with recurring gratitude and disbelief; through the next set of double doors; down a curving corridor; past the babies in single bays; into the pod for the sickest and smallest. Had I helped her or had I sentenced her? Had I been a mother to her at all?

Tracy had come in on her day off. I had a vision when I saw her. I was drowning in a churning ocean, choking on seawater and diesel fuel, unable to scream, and Tracy was a Dopplering light, a buoy tossed toward me in the wind.

Her only patient that day was Juniper, which meant a supervisor had calculated that things looked bad. I wanted to grab Tracy and beg for my baby's life. Instead I just scrubbed my hands.

As the water ran, I looked at my fingers. I had my mother's hands. She was seventy now and still worked in a hospital lab, refusing to retire. I pictured her in her white uniform, reaching to scoop me up after preschool. I felt her thumb, scratchy as the tongue of a cat, rubbing milk off my lip. A hospital lotion pump was mounted on the wall next to the soap. I skipped it. I wanted these rough, worn hands. I wanted to look at them and see evidence that I was someone's mom now, too.

"She had a great night," Tracy said. She was always careful not to let our expectations boomerang, but she told us she'd been surprised when she came in and saw that Juniper's blood pressure had stabilized, and that she required only 30 percent oxygen, down from 90.

"She's being a smart girl," Tracy said.

Diane and the surgeon stopped by. The surprise was visible on their faces, too.

"She's a tough little cookie," Diane said. "She's amazing."

Dr. Walford looked at the incision under the bandage and checked all the drains. She said she wouldn't even consider another surgery for at least a month, so there was nothing to do but wait and see.

"Why is it working?" I asked.

"Just go with it," Tracy said. "Enjoy the moment."

Maybe the simple act of cutting her open had relieved pressure in her abdomen, allowing her kidneys and lungs to function. Maybe one of the four soda-straw-size drains the surgeon had inserted in desperation had made a difference.

I texted Mike: *Tracy says to enjoy the moment.*

Mike: *Which moment? The terrifying one or the merely worrisome one?*

That afternoon, Dr. Shakeel stopped by Juniper's incubator, where Tom and I sat, waiting for something to happen and hoping that nothing did. I was curled, pale and fetal, in the narrow recliner. Dr. Shakeel pulled a chair close, leaned on her elbow, and looked at me. I couldn't remember another doctor doing that. I had forgotten that doctors could pause, or sit, or that they could see me at all.

"Babies are very, very resilient," she said. I just nodded. I stared off in the direction of the incubator. She was leaning in, and I was afraid her kindness was going to make me cry.

"I wish I could show you some of the babies," she said. "They pull out of it."

The doctors do what they can, she said, but the patient does the hardest work. Sometimes, when the surgeons think the cause is lost, the babies put themselves back together. Sometimes babies like Juniper, with holes in their guts, never even return to the operating room.

I had my chin in my hand and was rocking like a mental patient. I kept glancing at the doctor and back at my baby. Dr. Shakeel wrapped her arm around me.

"Where there's life," she told me, "there's hope."

When the doctor left, Tracy lifted the top off the incubator. She gently turned Juniper and nested her in a white blanket dotted with blue monkeys. She rolled and folded and tucked and smoothed until the baby had soft boundaries on every side, containing her, making her feel secure. I couldn't see the bottom half of Juniper's face, because of the tape and the wires. I couldn't see the bottom half of her belly, because of the bandages. But I was stunned that she could be so beautiful. She was asleep. Her hair swept sideways across her forehead over her arching eyebrows. Her hands were cuffed by bandages and IVs, but she tucked her little fists sweetly under her chin.

Her ears, which still contained no cartilage and held no shape, were scrunched against the blankets, so Tracy gently unfolded them. She left the top up on the incubator, inviting me to approach.

I decided to begin my own story vigil. On Kindle, I called up chapter 1 of *Winnie-the-Pooh*. I read to her about Pooh holding tight to the blue balloon, letting it carry him up, up, up off the ground and into the air, closer and closer to the honey in the tree, and how he convinced himself that he looked just like a cloud in the sky, and because of his cleverness the bees would never notice him, and he would reach the honey on the force of his stubborn hope, and he would never get stung. Until Christopher Robin said no, Pooh, you look like a bear holding a balloon.

Juniper survived the night.

The next day, we had a new nurse, Barbara, who evidently did not believe in sugarcoating.

Juniper's lungs were faltering again. Her ventilator settings were maxed out. She was on steroids to strengthen the lungs, but steroids can slow brain growth. They only gave steroids, Barbara said, to kids they thought would otherwise die. Juniper had been on them for some time.

I stared at this nurse and tried to interpret her report. Would my baby be stupid? Or merely have a small head? Was I grateful to her for leveling with me, or did I want to smack her in the mouth?

She kept on. She thought Juniper's chest was seizing up. "It's scary that she's doing that so young," she said. "Wow. Kids who do that are scary kids."

Tracy would be able to tell me if things were really this bad, but Tracy was off that day. Mike arrived for a visit. Tom headed downstairs to the cafeteria. Barbara, mercifully, stopped talking.

Mike and I watched while a respiratory therapist got ready to test Juniper's blood.

"Watch her numbers when he does this," I said to Mike.

The tech pricked her heel. Her oxygen saturation dived into the seventies; her heart rate dropped below one hundred. Alarms sounded.

"I just don't know how much longer I can feel this level of stress," I said. I had been hiding again. I had stayed home that day until almost four, afraid to disturb the bubble of calm in the quiet house. Some nights, I didn't even want to call the NICU to check on her. If this was all to punish me for wanting her so much, then if I wasn't at the hospital, if I didn't call, maybe nothing bad could happen to her. Maybe the curse was me.

"I'm afraid to open my eyes."

Mike said I needed to get away from the hospital. "I've got to think this is just really bad feng shui in here."

He was probably right. But what if she crashed while I was at Target or Taco Bus? What if these were our last hours together? How could I miss any of it? How would I ever know when it was safe? "I just wanted a baby," I said. "It's a common, normal thing to want."

"This isn't because of you," he said. "It's just random."

I didn't believe that. No one could be so unlucky. He was holding my hand now. I wondered if he would ever hold Juniper. If he did, she would feel so safe.

"She's *here*," he said. "Three weeks ago we didn't think we'd have that."

Yes, she was here. She was beautiful. She was a mirage. I couldn't hold her. I couldn't take her home. I just had to wait to find out if she was real.

"If this were a book," I said, "I would skip to the end."

"Listen," he said, "you can stand it. You are doing it. They are already throwing the worst at you every day."

"Almost the worst," I said.

"Almost the worst," he said, and we were quiet.

Juniper didn't die that day. She didn't die the next. She didn't die all that week. I was terrified that she'd die on Mother's Day, but she didn't. The holiday came and went, unacknowledged, even though I was fairly certain it was the only Mother's Day I'd ever have.

She didn't die, but in a way she disappeared. She bloated until she became unrecognizable. Her head grew misshapen, waterlogged. She couldn't move. She couldn't open her eyes. She was awful to look at. I didn't tell anyone this, but I'd delivered a stillborn puppy once who looked like her. The sight of it had scared me so much I'd wrapped it in a dish towel and stuffed it in a plastic bag. Now I had to find a way to reach my daughter, wherever she had gone.

Sitting stoop-shouldered on the swivel stool by her incubator, occupying the same few square feet of space that had been our cage for the past month, I tried to build a world for her out of pieces that didn't fit.

I talked to her about everything. I always started the same way. *Hi, beautiful. Mommy's here. I'm so proud of you.* She was sedated, so she never reacted. I was aware of the sound of my voice, of its rhythms and tone. I watched the monitor, but the clues were not there. I talked to God, too, but I did that in my head. I asked that Juniper have just one good day. She had lived more than a month, and each day had been measured in needle sticks, isolation, and pain. She'd been held only once. I didn't know if touching her brought her comfort or aggravation. I thought if she had one good day she would want one more, and another and another. Without that, what did she have to live for? Why would she fight?

Eventually I ran out of words. I picked up *Winnie-the-Pooh* and read about the Woozle and the Heffalump and the Expotition to the North Pole. I hoped that something in my voice, or in the cadence of the language, would comfort her.

It wasn't lost on me that the stories we chose carried messages of love and faith and friendship, and the shared experience of generations.

"A story is a promise," Tom had told me. "It's a promise that the end is worth waiting for."

I read to her about the great green room with the telephone

and the red balloon. As parents and children have done for decades, we invented new endings. "Good night, Dr. Shakeel. Good night, Tracy. Good night, IV pole. Good night, ventilator."

I finished *Winnie-the-Pooh* and *The House at Pooh Corner,* and when Piglet sidled up to Pooh and took his paw, I cried. I looked at my sleeping baby, and I read, "I just wanted to be sure of you."

Tom

Six days after the surgery, the team rolled Junebug and her incubator out of the pod and into a private room.

Room 670 was quiet and dark. We were secluded from the chorus of other babies' alarms. A row of thin windows ran along the top of the south wall but allowed in almost no sunshine. An overhead light hung above the incubator; usually it was switched off. The room was designed for hushed darkness. Our daughter was still two and a half months from her due date. Anything that encouraged her brain and body to develop as though she were still floating inside her mother could only help.

Always searching for coded messages, Kelley and I tried to interpret the move. Was it a good sign or an omen? Did the doctors believe Junebug no longer needed so many nurses hovering? Or did they want to give us privacy when she died?

"You guys are thinking too hard," Tracy said. "This room opened up, and you were next on the list."

No one on Junebug's medical team would predict whether she would ever leave Six South. The nurses grew uncomfortable if we broached the subject. False hopes would do us no good.

"These little ones," a nurse practitioner said one day, shaking her head as she gazed down at Junebug. "It doesn't take anything, and..."

She finished the thought with a wave of her hand, as though she were flicking away beads of water.

Junebug had survived her surgery, yes, but the surgery had not made her whole. The list of things that could kill her kept growing. The doctors weren't sure if her bowels were under attack from necrotizing enterocolitis. Her blood pressure kept dropping, and the doctors kept upping her dopamine, and still it would not stabilize. The threat of infection lingered. Her saturation level roller-coastered night and day. At rounds, Dr. Shakeel searched for answers.

"Is she desatting because of her lungs? Is she desatting because she's anemic? Why is she desatting?"

Junebug's head and body kept swelling. If it got much worse, the doctors worried, her stretching skin could pull open the stitches in her belly. She was a constellation of bruises. One thing everyone agreed on was that the surgery had left her in pain. Since newborns cannot talk, the nurses used a ten-point scale to assess their pain based on facial expressions and movements. A four was considered too high for a micro-preemie; Junebug's pain once spiked to an eight. The doctors increased her dosage of fentanyl, a narcotic more potent than morphine. Then someone explained that Junebug was addicted and would eventually have to be weaned. She would have to go through withdrawal, on top of everything else.

Junebug's latest X-rays had revealed a blood clot in her heart. Her PICC line had been pushed in too deep, and the clot had formed at the tip. The miscalculation had been easy enough to make, because everything inside her body was so small. Through bad luck, this clot had massed in one of the worst places possible. It was approximately six millimeters wide, big for a baby who still weighed less than two pounds. Tracy explained the problem.

"If it dislodges," she said, "that's dangerous."

"Dangerous?" I asked, pressing gently.

Tracy studied my face, deciding how much information I could handle.

"It could be fatal," she said.

Tracy explained that the PICC line had been pulled back, but the clot remained stuck to the wall of her right atrium, close to an opening that led to the left atrium. The doctors had ordered meds to dissolve the clot, but they were keeping the dosage low. If they rushed the problem, the meds might cause the clot to fracture, sending chunks drifting down the bloodstream toward her lung or brain. She could die in an instant.

When Tracy finished explaining, she studied me again.

"Does that help?" she said.

I nodded. Finally I was ready to learn. I had stopped spinning fairy tales in my head and the reporter in me was paying attention.

Junebug's complications were ghastly, but I wanted to understand them. I wanted to know everything about how the NICU worked and how the doctors made their calculations.

Over the weeks, I had watched different doctors adding up the same facts and arriving at fundamentally different conclusions. Dr. Shakeel, whom we adored and trusted, thought Juniper's intestines had burst simply because they were underdeveloped and weak. Another doctor, Joana Machry, worried they were under attack from necrotizing enterocolitis.

Dr. Machry had a soft voice and a kind face with big brown eyes that reminded me of a springer spaniel. Those eyes seemed especially misty when she painted the grim picture of what she feared might await us. In a few weeks, she said, when Junebug grew big enough for the surgeons to repair the damage, there was a chance that her intestines would already be dead.

The chasm between the diagnoses was confusing, yet it happened over and over. This doctor thought the swelling was caused by all of the fluids they were pumping into our daughter; that one thought it was a sign of infection. One person wanted to wean her off the oxygen quickly; another believed it was safer to move slowly.

At home, we pored through books and medical journals, and much of what we were learning was shocking. Neonatology, it turned out, had been built on devastating misjudgments: advances that were ignored or dismissed, lifesaving methods that were overlooked, the hasty introduction of medicines and treatments that had inadvertently hurt babies, or even killed them.

The first sputtering decades of neonatology were a massive improvement over the neglect of earlier times. For centuries, medicine devoted little attention to infants, leaving that responsibility to mothers. But in the 1800s, Europe's high infant mortality rate posed a problem. Fearing that it would run out of young workers and soldiers to expand its colonial empire, France opened maternity hospitals and special-care nurseries.

Stéphane Tarnier, France's chief obstetrician at the time, confessed to a colleague that he felt tortured when he arrived at Maternité Hospital in Paris on cold mornings and found many of the "weaklings" already gone still in their fleece cotton blankets. Then Tarnier visited the Paris zoo and admired a contraption designed to warm chicken eggs. The doctor asked the zookeeper who had created the device to adapt it for human babies.

Featuring more advanced models of incubators, the Pavillon des Délibes—Pavilion of Weaklings—was opened at Maternité in 1893. The pavilion staff treated 721 infants. Nearly half of them died, but at that point in France's history, a 51 percent survival rate stood as a remarkable improvement.

In the summer of 1896, another pavilion—the Kinderbrutanstalt, or Child Hatchery—opened in Berlin, featuring six incubators filled with prematurely born infants loaned from a nearby hospital. That exhibit was run by Dr. Martin Couney, a scientist and a showman, who would go on to display premature infants at several world's fairs. Couney's exhibits offered a level of care unmatched by any American hospital, but the medical establishment largely dismissed him.

Incubators were not widely used in the United States. They were expensive, and many physicians were unconvinced of their value. Some believed that premature babies were better left to die.

"These puny, ill-conditioned babies crowd out welfare stations and hospitals. Many of them die in later infancy," said Mary Mills West, the author of *Infant Care*, a manual distributed by the U.S. Children's Bureau, during a public address in 1915. "Still others live on, dragging out enfeebled existences, possibly becoming the progenitors of weaklings like themselves."

The eugenics movement took hold around the world. Some doctors allowed "defective" babies to die of starvation or neglect. Noting that a high percentage of premature babies were born to the poor, to minorities, and to immigrant families, some argued that intervening on behalf of these vulnerable newborns diluted the purity of American blood. Saving premature babies, these critics argued, was "race suicide."

Martin Couney's incubator shows offered refuge. An immigrant himself, Couney treated babies of all races and back-grounds. He never billed the parents. Instead, he met his high overhead by charging admission to his exhibits at fairs and amusement parks. At Chicago's Century of Progress Exposition, the incubator babies were located on the midway next to a burlesque show featuring Sally Rand, the famed fan dancer.

Couney settled into a permanent home at Coney Island. A lighted sign above the entrance proclaimed ALL THE WORLD LOVES A BABY. Carnival barkers roamed the boardwalk, luring customers with cries of "Don't pass the babies by!" Inside the exhibit, the atmosphere was quiet and clinical. Nurses stood guard in uniforms and white caps. Spectators, most of them women, paid a quarter to peer through glass at the living curiosities. Some returned again and again to watch the progress of one baby. Couney insisted he never solicited a child for one of his exhibits. All of them, he said, were brought to him by desperate parents or by hospitals and doctors who lacked the equipment and expertise to care for them. He bristled at the notion that he was running a freak show.

"All my life I have been making propaganda for the proper care of preemies," he said. "Everything I do is strictly ethical."

When A. J. Liebling caught up with Couney at the 1939 New York World's Fair for a *New Yorker* profile, the incubator doctor was contemplating retirement. His back was stooped. His hair and mustache had gone gray. He was having trouble meeting his overhead. But the crowds were still buying tickets to stare at his patients.

In the forty-three years since the Berlin exposition, Couney told Liebling, he and his nurses had cared for 8,000 preemies. Roughly 6,500 of them had been returned to their parents alive. Decades later, some of the survivors tracked Couney down to thank him. One of them was Lucille Horn, a graduate of the Coney Island exhibit. When she was born prematurely in 1920, weighing close to two pounds, the local hospital had refused to take her.

"They didn't have any help for me at all," she told her daughter on a visit with StoryCorps. "It was just: you die because you didn't belong in the world."

Horn's father knew where to take her. He wrapped her in a blanket, hailed a taxi, and headed for Coney Island.

"How do you feel knowing that people paid to see you?" her daughter asked.

"It's strange. But as long as they saw me and I was alive, it was all right," Horn answered. "Ninety-four years later, here I am, all in one piece."

Standing over Junebug's incubator, listening to the sighing of her vent, I could not help thinking about the origins of these machines. It was hard to fathom that so much of the technology had been developed to protect children destined to become cannon fodder.

At least the doctors who had invented incubators and ventilators had tried to do something. I imagined Dr. Tarnier on a winter's morning in Paris, making his rounds at Maternité Hospital and discovering that another newborn had died. I saw his face when he touched the cold skin. Between my fingers I felt the fabric of the fleece blanket as he pulled it up to cover the body. It was painful to think of all the losses that had fueled his determination. But I was grateful for the man and his work.

Inevitably, my mind returned to the boardwalk at Coney Island. I heard the carnival barkers and felt the heat of the lights, beckoning me inside to gawk. I paid my quarter and entered.

Through the glass, I saw the nurses scurrying, and the rows of incubators, hulking and primitive, vaguely resembling popcorn machines at movie theaters.

"What is an incubator?" Couney liked to say. "A peanut roaster."

In some of the black-and-white photos from the exhibits, the doctor and his nurses posed for the cameras, rocking their otherworldly patients in their arms, often two at a time. Peering from their blankets were the same scrunched homunculus faces I had glimpsed in the delivery room when Junebug was pulled into the light. None of Couney's babies were as small. In those days, the outer limit of viability was roughly thirty weeks gestation. But when I studied the photos, gazing across the arc of a century, I saw my daughter in each of them.

Had Junebug been born prematurely back then, would Kelley and I have wrapped her in a warm blanket and hurried her to Coney Island, knowing strangers would stare at our little girl like a freak?

In a second.

Kelley

Diane folded back the quilt covering Juniper's incubator and opened the portholes.

"Oh, little girl," she said, "little girl, little girl."

It was mid-May, about a week and a half after the failed surgery. Under the gauze on Juniper's stomach, the incision was a jagged gray gash. The drains placed by the surgeon had worked their way out, and the holes had scabbed over, but we wouldn't know for a few weeks whether her intestines had healed. The doctors had warned us of scarring and blockages and, in the worst case, dead sections of her gut. She would need more surgery later. As Dr. Machry had told us, babies who go through this sometimes don't have enough healthy intestine left to survive. Doctors had a name for it: short gut.

Short gut. Short stuff. Short bus. It was too fucking much.

Diane probed Juniper's brown, distended belly, checking for firmness that would indicate pressure inside. It was soft. That was good. With a little square of gauze, she wiped the scab on the right side where one of the drains had been. Out came a dab of strange green goop. This was bizarre. She wiped again. More goop.

A horrifying breach had opened in our baby's plumbing. It was poop, Diane said. Coming from a place where poop should not be.

I couldn't even think.

"Little one, little one, little one," Diane said.

As always, Diane was outwardly calm. She considered the situation for a moment, and then she told us it could even be a positive development. Had the surgery been successful, the surgeon would have created an escape hatch just like this in order to give Juniper's lower intestines a rest. The surgery had essentially failed, but in the days since, Juniper's body had rerouted itself through what was called a fistula. Poop was oozing out the most convenient exit, the way smoke works its way out of a cave. Diane said they would attach a little ostomy bag to the hole under her ribs and add the new plumbing problem to the list of things to fix later.

I was too numb to panic, but I did wonder if she was making that up. Feces leaking from our baby's belly did not seem right. Maybe our daughter had erupted inside, and Diane didn't want to tell us that this was how death came, even for babies— in filth and stench and shit.

Diane kept working, quietly. She noticed that Juniper had grown. She weighed almost two pounds, but so much of that was fluid from the swelling, it was hard to guess her real weight. Diane brushed back Juniper's hair with her fingertips, so gently, and touched what she could of her face, between the tubing and the tape.

Juniper was still too swollen to open her eyes. When we held her hand, she barely gripped back. She'd begun to twitch and jerk, signs of withdrawal from the pain medications. We had made her an addict. Yet taking her off the pain meds too abruptly would have been cruel. They continued to drip silently into her IV.

"I want to ask you a hard question," Tom said to Diane.

"Remember how that very first day we met you, you said there were some parents who pushed for the staff to keep working on their baby even beyond the point where it made any sense?"

Diane nodded.

"Well, have we become those people?"

It surprised me that he asked it. I was usually the blunt one. But it was impossible not to wonder. The questions were so immense and so immediate. All you had to do was glance around, take in the sheer number of babies, all of them silent, gripping their little ventilator tubes, sedated into stillness. They couldn't voice an opinion about whether their lives were worth living. In front of us was our daughter, with her lumpy, sodden head, who couldn't tell us how much pain was too much. Medical progress was dazzling. But was all of this for her, or for us?

Diane shook her head. No, we hadn't yet pushed her too far. "Not even close," she said. "But I'll tell you if we reach that point."

She didn't tell us that some of her colleagues, seeing our baby go on and off the oscillating ventilator, seeing her wheeled to surgery and back, seeing her swell and bloat, seeing her oxygen settings rise precariously, had sidled up to her and whispered the same question. *Do the parents still want everything done?*

"Everything done" was NICU shorthand. We didn't really comprehend what it entailed. We wanted the ventilator, because she couldn't breathe. We wanted intravenous nutrition, because she couldn't eat. We wanted all the interventions that could still leave her with a chance at a good life. But if her heart stopped, would we ask them to perform CPR? Some parents did, again and again, as tiny ribs cracked. We did not want that for her.

What she wanted for herself, we couldn't know. Most

humans hooked up to this level of machinery were elderly, capable of weighing in, of saying yes to CPR but no to dialysis. Juniper couldn't tell us if she'd had enough or what amount of disability she could accept. We thought she was showing a determination to fight, but maybe that was just blind hope.

Sometimes, doctors and parents clashed over the best course for a baby. Parents have sued hospitals for wrongful life as well as wrongful death. They have sued for saving babies like Juniper against their wishes and leaving them to care for profoundly disabled children. They have sued for refusing to resuscitate babies as young as twenty-one weeks, babies the medical community would universally agree had no chance at meaningful life. Every doctor and nurse knew the agony of trying to jolt life back into a baby who was too broken to save. One father of a twenty-five-weeker, himself a dermatologist, removed his baby's ventilator with his own hands.

There was no clear legal mandate, and I was glad for that. The last thing any of us needed was meddling politicians. We asked one doctor, Roberto Sosa, what happened when doctors and parents disagree. Dr. Sosa had founded the NICU at All Children's, and it was obvious he'd long thought about the question.

"Sometimes," he said, "the baby decides."

He told a story about a baby born even smaller than Juniper. The parents had decided to let the baby go. They had wanted him very much, but now that they'd made their choice, they couldn't bear to look at him. The staff agreed, kept the baby warm, and waited for him to die.

Morning came, and as Dr. Sosa was arriving at the office and hanging up his coat, his phone rang. It was Dr. Shakeel, the neonatologist on duty. The baby was pink and crying, she told him. The little guy had hung on all night, with no ventilator, no food, not even water. Now the hospital faced a moral obligation—and maybe a legal one—to help him. The baby was asserting his will, but the parents had made up their minds, and it was too painful to consider that their choice might have been the wrong one. The father told the doctors, "No one better go near my baby."

"You need to come over here and help me," Dr. Shakeel told Dr. Sosa.

The two doctors eventually persuaded the mother to look at her son. When she saw her baby she cried, "Save him!"

The baby grew big and healthy in the NICU. The nurses nicknamed him Stuart Little and fitted him with a tiny pair of roller skates from a key chain.

"The cutest little thing on the unit," recalled Dr. Shakeel.

"He was perfect," said Dr. Sosa. "Perfect."

Even if Tom and I had been at our best, the calculations were wrenching. But we were shattered versions of ourselves, handicapped by sleep deprivation and panic. No lawyer's form could protect us. We had only these kind people in their white coats. I trusted some more than others, but even that was absurd. If they made eye contact, remembered my child's name, smiled, spoke with confidence, I would consent to whatever they asked.

Here came one now. Dr. Carine Stromquist was one of my favorites, a slip of a woman with a light Belgian accent. She was neither arrogant nor insecure. She made time to explain things.

Diane showed her the smear of poop on the gauze.

"Here's what I wiped off."

"Mmmm."

They talked about clots and pressors and cortisol and albumin. Juniper needed meds for blood pressure, but more meds meant more fluids entering her body, exacerbating the leaking of her blood vessels and the drop in her blood pressure and the swelling. The swelling squeezed her lungs and heart. Dr. Stromquist wanted to wean her off the ventilator, to spare her lungs; wean the sedatives to help with the swelling; supplement with proteins to counteract the steroids; pump in albumin to draw fluid out of her tissues; try to make her pee more, breathe more, move more.

"It's a slow process," Dr. Stromquist said.

Diane wanted to wean her off some of the antibiotics, too.

"We don't know what we're treating," Diane said. "All her cultures are negative. All of them. I think we're chasing our tails."

I struggled to follow it all, but the scenario shifted by the hour. Every player had a different theory. Lost in the minutiae of intake and output was the real question: Was she going to live?

That night, I read to her from Tina Fey's book, the chapter she writes as a prayer for her daughter. May she grow up beautiful but not damaged; may the Lord lead her away from acting but not all the way to finance; may she play drums, with her own power and rhythm, so she need not lie with drummers. The prayer took on an extra measure of faith there in that darkened room.

The alarm sounded. Maybe Juniper didn't want anyone telling her whom she could or could not date.

"Come on up, baby," I said, watching the sat number tick upward. "That's a good girl."

The number rose, then fell again.

Our nurse, Kim Jay, listened from the corner of the room, where she sat at a computer, updating the chart.

"She's teasing us," she said.

When Kim opened the incubator to check on her that night, Juniper forced open a swollen eye and peeked out.

Tom

I woke with a start in the middle of a Saturday night, fighting to climb out of the pit of another harrowing dream. The details slipped away the moment I opened my eyes, but the foreboding still gripped me so tightly that at first I was not sure I was awake. For a minute or two, I stared up at the ceiling fan and listened to the hum of its blades spinning in the dark and waited for the mad thumping in my chest to slow.

I reached for my phone on the shelf behind the bed and called the hospital.

"Room Six-seventy, please."

Kelley was asleep beside me. We were starting to hold hands again, and sometimes when I drove, she would reach over and brush her fingers on my cheek. But most of the time she still felt far away.

On the other end of the line, someone picked up.

"NICU, this is Kim."

I felt better when Kim Jay was on duty. She was our primary nurse on the night shift, a veteran who knew as much about preemies as anyone on the floor.

"How's she doing?" I asked.

"She's having a good night," Kim said. "Very quiet."

Her voice was calm, with a hint of playfulness. During my

216

late-night check-ins, I often had the impression that my daughter had just taken out her vent to tell a joke and that Kim was not quite done laughing. But when we hung up, my anxiety returned. The moment I closed my eyes, I fell back into the pit.

When I awoke again, it was just after four, and I could not shake the certainty that something irreversible was happening inside Junebug. Something had been going wrong for days, and no one knew it, and now she was bursting.

Outside, a lightning strike lit the sky. I blinked, and as the flash faded and then surged again, I caught an electric snapshot of our backyard. Then came the depth charge of thunder, growling in the distance, and the rain falling against the roof in waves. The storm had been building for some time, and I realized that I had heard the lightning and thunder in my nightmare. But understanding this did not make my dread go away.

I headed for the hospital at dawn. By then the storm had washed the sky so clear that from the interstate I could just make out the Tampa skyline across the bay. The sun was painting the horizon with swaths of pink and orange and purple, like a massive canvas dreamed up by Rothko.

As I walked into All Children's, I passed the usual parade of moms and dads, pale and bleary-eyed, clutching pillows and blankets as they staggered toward the garage. On the other floors of the hospital, parents often stayed overnight in the rooms. I marveled at their resilience. They had sat up beside their kids through the night, listening to them talking fitfully in their sleep and absorbing the monitor alarms and replaying every quiet conversation with the hospital chaplain, and now they had to stumble back to work and act as though they still had a life outside this building. How did they do it?

When I arrived in the room, Junebug was struggling. Her

swelling had not stopped, and the back of her head was so engorged that it bulged like a block. Her eyes were shut, and she barely moved, except for a jerking in her arms. She didn't want to be touched. She hadn't had a good day since the surgery. When I held her hand, her grip was weak. Under all the swelling, the little girl we knew was morphing into a mere receptacle for tubes and wires and lines, a vessel for all the doctors' protocols and procedures.

I was fighting not to lose it when Dr. McCarthy walked in. I hadn't seen her since the day my daughter was born, when her wizened face and all-knowing aura had reminded me of Yoda. On that day, her presence had reassured me. Now I didn't know what to think. Why was she making this surprise appearance?

"Everything looks good, except I'm wondering about the swelling in her head," Dr. McCarthy said. "I'm not sure why that's happening."

She opened the incubator and reached in to gently turn Junebug's head. She checked her oxygen and her meds and then looked at the baby's head again. She seemed preoccupied with the mystery of the swelling, and more anxious than she wanted to let on. She listed possible causes for the extra fluid and explained that she had ordered an ultrasound to see if the baby's PICC was leaking. The silences between the doctor's sentences seemed long and heavy with implication.

By now I was picking up nuances about the NICU that weren't in the brochure. I had learned some of the secret language of the floor, from the receptionist to the elders. I had seen them make their offerings to ward off evil spirits, had noted what made them laugh and what made them angry, the knowing glances they exchanged when they thought no one was watching. I had witnessed the rituals they observed at dawn and their quiet midnight gatherings as they fought to save another life. I knew what their faces looked like when they were succeeding, the way their jaws set when they accepted that nothing more could be done.

The snippets I'd caught from Yoda were chilling.

The dread stayed with me all day. When I couldn't stand it anymore, I went to Publix to scrounge something for dinner. I had just gotten home and was putting away the groceries when All Children's called. Junebug's swelling was worse, and her blood pressure was dropping, and her urine output was meager, and she might be fighting an infection. They were taking blood and urine cultures. They were putting in a new catheter. They also wanted to replace her PICC line, a procedure complicated enough that they needed our permission before proceeding. They wanted one of us to come down immediately.

Kelley was worried and frustrated, because she was feeling a scratch in her throat and thought she might be getting sick. She couldn't risk infecting Junebug. I gave her a kiss and hurried out the door.

On the way in, I remembered the nightmare, the lightning and the thunder, the foreboding that had gripped me in the night and clung to me all day. My subconscious had gathered all the cues I was picking up during my waking hours and had analyzed the evidence and sent me a message of startling simplicity.

Juniper was exploding.

When I walked in, Yoda was standing by the incubator, looking even more concerned than before. She was upping the baby's hydrocortisone, she said, due to her "adrenal insufficiency." I didn't know exactly what that meant, but it was obviously connected to getting Junebug's blood pressure up.

"I don't know why she's having trouble holding her blood pressure," said Dr. McCarthy. "It could be just that she's so small that her kidneys simply aren't adjusting yet."

A nurse and lab tech were taking the cultures from her blood and urine and prepping her for the catheter. They'd covered her face with gauze and swabbed her groin with Betadine, and now the tech was holding my daughter's legs open and clearing away all the lines going into her body, so nothing would get tangled or yanked.

"You got her peripheral?" said the nurse as she moved in close.

"I got her peripheral," said the tech.

"All right, girlie," said the nurse, shining a light as she tried to insert the catheter.

But it wouldn't go in. The catheter was too big for Junebug's urethra.

Even though the nurse was gripping her legs, and even though her body was so swollen that she almost could not move, Junebug was somehow managing to writhe and kick and thrash. It was the only way she could scream.

"I'm so sorry, baby," said the nurse.

"I don't blame her," said the tech.

I held my breath and prayed for it to stop.

"That's a five, right?" said the tech, wondering if they had the wrong-size tube.

More kicking.

"Yeah."

More straining and thrashing. She was doing anything she could to get away from them.

220

"You might need a three-point-five."

She was desatting now, silently screaming on and on, and I could not help her. In my head I was begging them to stop, to go get the fucking 3.5 or whatever they needed so they could please, please, please stop hurting my baby. Finally they got the line inside her. Even then, as they closed up her diaper, she kept thrashing. I could barely stand it. Was the line so big that it was still hurting her?

"I know, girl," said the nurse.

They weren't done. Once the catheter was in, another team arrived to put in the new PICC line. This was why they'd had me sign the consent form. The procedure was sensitive enough that the NICU did not allow parents to witness it, so they asked me to leave. But before I walked out, the charge nurse told me that they were putting Junebug back on the fentanyl drip. The thought of it made me wince.

I dropped into a chair in the family lounge. The TV was blaring with an adventure show for kids. A character obviously modeled after Indiana Jones, down to the hat, was leaping and running and overemoting in rapid-fire Spanish. I ignored it and gazed out the window toward the light-blue vault of the sky arching over the dark blue of the water. It was the same vista I'd admired early that morning, only now sunset was coming and everything was bathed in the falling light.

Night would be here soon. Maybe Junebug would sleep. Maybe both of us would.

I was still staring out the window, watching the sky deepen toward violet, when I looked at my phone and realized I'd been sitting here for more than an hour. I couldn't understand why no one had called me to say the procedure was over and I could return to the room. The last time they'd put a PICC into

Junebug, the nurses had only asked me to leave for fifteen minutes or so. Why was this time taking so much longer?

I stood up and headed back into the unit, so I'd be closer when they called. I found a seat on a couch near the front reception desk and began listening to the older woman answering the phones. She was hard to ignore, because she had a big bubbly voice reined in by a German accent. Whenever the phone rang, she reminded me of a grandmother in combat boots.

"NICU!" she'd say, stretching out the *U* until it sang. "Hansi!"

Hansi's voice was loud enough that I could hear everything she was saying to a younger woman sitting beside her. They were reviewing which nurses were assigned that night to which babies, and Hansi was commenting on the abundance of Sarahs on the nursing staff. I appreciated the way Hansi was occupying my mind. An hour and a half had gone by, and still there was no word from the PICC team. I focused on the receptionist's voice, the operatic rhythms of her sentences, the sudden flights that accompanied each exclamation point, the way her accent gave her perkiness a militaristic edge.

"NICU! Hansi!" A pause. "Linda down in X-ray, what can I do for you?"

A longer pause while she listened.

"Okey-dokey."

An even longer pause.

"If I make a boo-boo sometimes," she said, "it's made with tons of love."

In the middle of this small talk, I heard something that made my heart stop.

"Should I make a minimum of labels," Hansi was saying to the young woman beside her, "just in case this baby doesn't survive?"

"Yes," said the other woman, lowering her voice.

Though they never uttered the name of the baby in question, I suspected they were talking about Junebug. Maybe the procedure had gone wrong. Maybe the team was back in the room now, debating who would get the awful task of coming out to inform me that my daughter was dead. Even if that were true, I couldn't figure out how Hansi or the other woman would already know. Was everyone on the staff alerted when a baby was close to the edge? Did word travel instantly around the floor?

My heart was back to its thumping. Again I searched for a focal point. I listened to the hum of the air-conditioning, the sounds of the elevator doors opening and closing, the faint and familiar cry from inside the elevators.

"Going down!"

As I weighed the evidence on whether my daughter was dead, someone else walked up to the front desk to tell Hansi about her weekend. She'd had fun. There were pictures of the fun.

"I love photos!" Hansi cried.

The other person wandered away, and Hansi began to hum one of those marches you hear on the Fourth of July. I was pretty sure it was John Philip Sousa's "Stars and Stripes Forever." She was doing the brass parts by pursing her lips and blowing out the tune.

I couldn't help laughing to myself, but I did not know if I was laughing because this woman was so funny or because I had reached the end. If Junebug was dead, I would always associate this moment with Hansi's trumpet imitation. If Junebug was alive, I would invite Hansi over for a barbecue and ask her to repeat her performance. I mean, she had a gift.

The phone rang.

"NICU, Hansi!"

She listened for a few seconds and then called out.

"Mr. French? You can go back now."

It was 6:47 p.m., almost exactly two hours since they'd begun the procedure. Inside the room, Junebug was asleep. The day nurse was gone. The charge nurse was gone. The only evidence of whatever had happened was a swab stick on the floor, stained with blood.

I nearly cried when I saw Kim sitting in the corner, updating the chart as she began another night shift. She told me that the procedure had failed. They'd tried to put a new line in one of Junebug's legs, but they couldn't make it work. Then they tried to put one in her other leg, with the same result. The team would have to wait a few days and give it another shot. Kim was letting Junebug sleep. I walked over to my girl and whispered a few words to her so that maybe, somewhere deep down, she would know I was there.

In the room across the hall, a baby yelled from inside his incubator. His nurse tried to shush him, but her attentions only ramped up the volume of his protests.

"Holy smokes," said the nurse. "You're crazy, you know that?"

Kelley

Every day that she didn't die made it easier to believe that she might not, but the evidence was there in her medical chart.

> *Grossly edematous*
> *Worsening opacities bilaterally*
> *Rarely has spontaneous respiratory effort*

On her thirty-seventh day of life, I turned thirty-seven years old, and I got to hold her again. A gift from the nurses.

I watched the team in their elaborate, slow-motion maneuvering to move her onto my chest. In the tiny space between the incubator and the recliner, it looked like a tango in a coat closet. If Ana Maria stumbled, and Juniper arced through the air, trailing her wires, tripping her alarms, would I have the reflexes to catch her?

She weighed twice what she had the first time — a whole two and a half pounds. It was just the swelling, of course. Water weight. Even as bloated as she was, I could cover her whole back with the length of my fingers. She felt like a small pigeon.

How did she make sense of me? Did she have memory, or just some primal recognition? I tried to freeze time. Tracy had stuck a purple bow on her head and a little tattoo on her chest — "I ♥ Mom" on clear tape. The accessorizing failed to obscure the obvious. She had lived five weeks, and it seemed she had been dying the entire time.

"We've got to get this fluid off her," Diane said.

She was so swollen that the fluid leaked out of her skin, beading on the surface like sweat. She'd plumped like a baking biscuit. Her neck had disappeared, and her forehead bulged into a fat wrinkle above her nose. I had stopped taking pictures of her. If she lived, I didn't want her to see herself this way. If she died, I didn't want to remember her like this.

For days, the doctors debated what to do about the swelling. Fluid was part of the body's response to injury. The vessels opened so antibodies and coagulants could leach through to the source of the damage. Blood pressure dropped, blood couldn't carry waste to the kidneys, and poisons built up.

I stared at her, fat and dewy in her blankets, while they talked about dry weights and drips.

"This will sound dumb, I guess," I said one morning at rounds. "But if this were my cell phone, and I had dropped it in the pool, I'd put it in a bag of rice. Can we just lay her on a bed of rice?"

Tom nervous-laughed like *Oh, don't mind my wife, she's under a lot of stress.*

The nurses pumped albumin into her IV to pull fluid back into her vessels. They pumped in Lasix to force her to pee. They pumped in dopamine to boost her blood pressure. The pole next to her bed that held the pumps for the various medicines grew overloaded, so they wheeled in a second one.

All those medicines needed an avenue into her body, but access, as the nurses called it, was a constant struggle. The little IVs you get in your hand or arm for an overnight stay at the hospital don't hold long. When patients linger in the hospital for months, nurses need a pipeline to the fat central veins in the torso and neck. Because of Juniper's busted gut, her nutrition, lipids, and meds were all flowing into her bloodstream. It was a lot for a little person to absorb, and some medicines couldn't mix in the same vein.

When they looked for a new point of entry, they would shine a flashlight underneath her arm, lighting all the way through her skin. The veins in her arm showed squirrelly and squiggly as they jagged around the scarring from previous needle sticks.

The situation was making Tracy tense. I watched her as she examined this arm, that leg, even Juniper's head.

"Did you find a spot?" I asked.

"I'm still looking," Tracy said, peering over her mask. "It's not finding a spot, it's finding the best spot. She doesn't have a lot of those left."

Juniper's oxygen dropped to seventy-two. Her toes were curling and uncurling.

"Be a good girl, give me a bigger vein," Tracy said. "Don't be bashful."

Tracy wanted a catheter called a Broviac to ferry the goods straight to the doorway of Juniper's heart. That meant summoning the reluctant surgeon again. Tracy, with her cool midwestern pragmatism, impressed on Dr. Walford the importance of planning ahead. She urged her to put in the Broviac now, before an emergency struck.

"I'd hate to have to call you on a Sunday," Tracy said.

The catheter went in.

Juniper needed a break. Finally, near the end of May, she got one. The doctors figured out that keeping her blood pressure over fifty-five would make her pee. All babies were different, Dr. Stromquist explained, and Juniper was finicky about her blood pressure. So they manipulated the meds, and mercifully, the swelling began to go down.

In a matter of days, she looked more like a baby. She looked more like a baby than she ever had, because now she had matured. It was as though our daughter had been forming in a place we could not see, and when the swelling went down, a new person appeared.

She still had no body fat, so as she shrank, she again took on the dimensions of an old man, with spindly arms and legs and knobby knees. Her face had softened, though, and her eyes opened into dark pools. She looked around quizzically, her eyebrows arching with the effort. She was curious and aware. Her tiny fists clenched and unclenched around her ventilator tube. She was no longer content to lie inert in the bed. She tried to turn her head from side to side, to see what was going on, but the tube kept her anchored. The nurses had to make sure to use plenty of tape, because they didn't want her to pull the thing out.

Tracy became emboldened in her accessorizing. She fashioned a bow out of zebra fabric and pink ribbon that was so comically large I started referring to it as the Aretha Franklin inauguration hat. Aretha's gray-felt headgear, with the enormous, tilted rhinestone-rimmed bow, stole Obama's inauguration in 2009. Now it resided in the Smithsonian and toured with the Rock and Roll Hall of Fame, and a baby in Florida wore a tiny tribute.

I'd heard that Tracy had a reputation for preemie pranks, but with us she had shown restraint. Maybe this cartoonish bow meant Juniper was no longer so close to the edge. One morning at Cracker Barrel, I passed a display of Christmas ornaments—in late spring, mind you—shaped like tiny musical instruments. I picked up a red electric guitar with wire strings, four inches long. The next morning, I propped it in Juniper's arms. A perfect fit.

Tracy turned around and saw and laughed, and something inside her broke free.

The annual All Children's Telethon was approaching. The organizers had asked to feature Juniper, but Dr. Yoda vetoed it. Juniper's prognosis was still too grim. Instead, she would get a few seconds of airtime as the camera crew roamed incubator to incubator down preemie row, assuring viewership, and hopefully donations, by so many grandmas. Pimpin' the Preemies, the nurses called it. Tracy put Juniper in the tiniest dress, maybe six inches from top to bottom, with black-and-white stripes and a pink tulle skirt. Instantly, I knew photos of this first outfit would haunt her in the middle-school years.

"Where'd you get that dress?" I asked Tracy.

"The pet aisle," she said. "It's for Chihuahuas."

Thereafter, Tracy and I kept her outfitted in grand style, from places like Lil Yorkie Fru Fru and Doggie Diva Boutique. Not only were the dog dresses hilarious and tiny, but the Velcro collars and open backs made dressing her a snap and left plenty of room for the wires. On my afternoons, I stopped off at dog boutiques I had once mocked. I'd had no idea Chihuahuas dressed so well. I couldn't afford half of what I saw. Most of the ensembles were still too big for Juniper. Even in canine sizes, she wore an XXS.

When I entered one store, a gaggle of blue-haired ladies greeted me as they sat around watching "Real Housewives" and sipping white wine.

"What kind of dog do you have?" one of them asked.

"Oh, it's not for a dog," I said. "It's for a baby."

"Oh yes. They are our babies, aren't they, dear?"

"No, really," I said. "It's for a human baby. My dog is a pit bull, and she wouldn't be caught dead in any of this."

We were having fun, but it felt like tempting fate. Juniper looked better, but she was still awfully sick. She still needed the ventilator, and pretty soon X-rays showed why. Her lungs appeared hazy and white, indicating that fluid was pooling around them. The fluid made it hard for her to breathe, as if she were buried in sand.

"It's always something, cutie-pie," her nurse Cindy said one morning in late May.

"She's not going to give me a quiet day," Dr. Stromquist said.

"She's a puzzle," Diane said.

Diane inserted a needle between her ribs on each side and drew out the strange, clear fluid by the teaspoonful. Eventually, she put in chest tubes attached to a bubbling suction machine that sounded like a water feature at a spa. A half-cup of fluid or more poured out, day after day. The tubes hurt if they were jostled, so we wouldn't be able to hold her until they came out. I watched the yellowish liquid snake through the tubing into a bag and tried to pretend I was meditating next to a babbling brook.

Through experimentation the doctors learned that fats in her diet made the fluid turn cloudy. That meant that somehow she had a rupture in her lymphatic system. Of all the systems in the body, this surely was the one I had thought about the least. I had to consult Google to understand what it did. Turns out it's like a second circulatory system that carries white blood cells around your body. It cleans up toxins and fights infections. It also delivers some types of fats from your digestive tract to cells that need them.

Sometimes when people have chest surgery, the lymphatic system gets nicked by a scalpel or a probe. Some people are born with faulty ducts. Neither of those scenarios applied to Juniper, but there it was anyway. She had a weird condition called chylothorax, and no one knew why. It was not a common micro-preemie thing. It was not in the litany of calamities Dr. Germain had warned us about. It was freakish and unlucky.

Diane wondered if the lymphatic channel in her abdomen had gotten plugged, causing fluid to back up in her chest. Dr. Stromquist thought it could be related to an old clot on one of her central lines. Or maybe, like everything else, that part of her was just underdeveloped and it broke. No one said explicitly that chylothorax could kill her, but she couldn't live with it either.

"What the heck is going on with this girl?" Tracy said. "I'm going to have to give her a stern talking-to."

Soon it was June, and our daughter was two months old. We hugged Dr. Shakeel good-bye and greeted a new doctor, our third. They rotated every few weeks, because the most critical cases were hard on them, too. As much as I loved Dr. Shakeel, I didn't really care if she needed a break. She knew my baby best, and I wanted her to stay. I was crushed. Everyone was coming and going except us.

Dr. Rajan Wadhawan was our new neonatologist. The nurses called him Dr. Raj. He was calm and assertive, quick to smile. He sat down with us to review Juniper's progress. It felt like our first parent-teacher conference. When a baby was very sick, the doctors and nurses would say it was not behaving. We'd had a bad baby for a long time.

We perched on swivel chairs in a cramped office off the NICU as Dr. Raj methodically reviewed the obstacles Juniper faced, in order of urgency. The most pressing concern was the blood clot that lingered in her heart. If a piece broke loose, it could still slalom through her vessels until it reached her lung or her brain and killed her.

Some days, a full cup of fluid poured from the tubes in her chest. Dr. Raj called it the most confounding case of chylothorax he had seen. It meant Juniper couldn't be fed the breast milk I was still torturing myself to produce, because the fats in the milk exacerbated the problem. In a day or so, they'd start giving her a foul concoction through a tube, testing her healing gut.

Next came the scarring in her lungs from the ventilator, her mind-of-their-own intestines, and the constant threat of infection. She was getting too few calories and growing too slowly. Her kidneys and liver were stressed.

Death remained a real possibility. So did blindness, deafness, cerebral palsy, and an array of developmental delays. So did life on a feeding tube or on oxygen.

I still clung to an image of a little girl holding my hand on the way to kindergarten. She would try to hide her nerves as she bounced on her toes, thrilled with her new big-girl backpack and sparkly boots. I could remember my own mom taking me to kindergarten. I could remember clinging to her neck, the crispness of her hospital uniform under my cheek.

"Just one more question," I asked Dr. Raj. "Could she still be a normal kid?"

Dr. Raj shifted into analytics. He explained that on that question, statistics were lacking. It was hard to do certain kinds of research on fragile human infants. The logistical, legal, and ethical concerns were mind-boggling. When it came to babies as small as Juniper, it was hard to find enough of them for a big study. And technology evolved so fast that by the time a NICU kid reached middle school and someone noted his progress and wrote it up in a journal, the treatments and prospects for that year's crop of newborns had already changed.

Research did point to a few key indicators of how a child would turn out. The first was whether they had suffered a serious brain bleed. Juniper had not. Point for Juniper! But there were other factors, including what happened with her lungs, eyes, and intestines, and we didn't have all of those answers yet. It all added up to maybe.

I thought back to that early conversation with Dr. Germain, where he had laid out the grim probabilities. Again I wanted to interrogate the researchers, but it was no use. Then Dr. Raj said something profound. He said that the most important indicator of how a child fared was the environment in which they grew up. Parents, he said, mattered even more than whether the babies had bled inside their brains.

Neonatologists follow babies until they leave the hospital, but they usually don't see their patients as toddlers or first-graders. As many as half of former micro-preemies need help in school in the early years, studies show, but they do tend to catch up as they get older. The brain recovers from its perilous start. Time was a big part of the equation, but the biggest difference maker was whether the child had two parents, whether they grew up poor or comfortably middle-class, and whether their mom had a solid education.

Juniper had two working parents with four college degrees between them. She had her own room in a cozy, three-bedroom, two-bath home mortgaged with a reasonable interest rate. Point. Point. Point for Juniper. I'd been struggling to find my place, feeling helpless and overwhelmed. Now Dr. Raj was telling us, in his authoritative, backed-with-numbers, white-coated way, that we mattered.

The conversation was so different from the one we had had with Dr. Shakeel. "Where there's life, there's hope," she had said. She had been pure heart that day, and now Dr. Raj was helping us understand the science. We needed both—the structure of the research, and the faith and compassion of the people who interpreted it.

Tom

The NICU was swallowing me. I was haunted by the notion that Junebug could die ten minutes after I stepped away, so I lingered. Most days I was in her room at sunrise so I could talk to her and read to her and hear the doctors' daily forecast at rounds, and then I'd be back again in the afternoon, and again at night, sometimes until I nodded off in the chair. The nurses who didn't know me couldn't figure out if I was unemployed or just irresponsible.

"Where do you work again?" they'd ask. "Doesn't your boss wonder where you are?"

Tracy understood that I had no shortage of time off, at least until classes started back up in late August. That didn't mean she thought it was a great idea for me to live in Six South.

"You need to get out of here," she told me. "Otherwise you're going to crash, and that won't be good for you or Kelley or Junebug."

I could feel myself fraying. I began ducking out every day after rounds. Most of the time Kelley was still pumping her milk at home, so I'd head for Banyan. Sometimes Roy joined me, but if Junebug was having an extra-bad day, I went alone and sat at the counter and tried to settle into some semblance of calm.

Erica, the lovely woman who owned Banyan, could tell if I

needed quiet, and on those days she brought me a cappuccino in a big yellow Fiestaware mug and one of Banyan's breakfast sandwiches without me having to say a word. The sandwiches came on crisp Cuban bread that Erica had bought fresh that morning, and the egg was always fried somewhere between easy and medium, and the bacon was thick and crunchy, and I don't know how he did it every day, but the guy who made the sandwiches back in the tiny kitchen—his name was Rich—always sprinkled on just the right amount of salt and pepper, and when Erica brought it out and placed it before me on a thick Fiesta plate, the sandwich was still so hot that I could barely hold it, which was exactly what I liked.

Once, when Kelley and I were doing some couples counseling, the therapist asked us to name the place we each felt safest. When it was my turn, I answered instantly.

"The booth at Banyan."

The booth had deep benches and a wooden-slab table lit by a picture window. Roy called it Poets Corner because it had a shelf of books and a big blackboard where you could write quotes from your favorite author. Often I filled it with Springsteen lyrics. Roy and I liked to sit there and talk about whatever we were writing and whatever we were reading while we gazed out the window and watched homeless people peeing without shame on the live oaks across the street.

What truly set Banyan apart was Erica and her ever-revolving crew. They were ever-revolving because Erica was always firing them. She was nice about it, but she swung her ax so frequently that back in the kitchen they recorded the names of all the people she had terminated, some of whom had been rehired only to be dismissed yet again. The death list, they called it. Once, she had fired a server at the start of her first shift, after Erica saw her eating a free meal before she'd waited on a single table. On the death list, as the cause of her termination, the kitchen staff wrote "Hungry." Erica banished unruly customers, took away their food, found subtle ways to punish lesser offenses. She stocked the restaurant with virtually every color of Fiestaware, but she hated the light purple known as Plum, and whenever she served someone on a Plum plate, that was her way of signaling disdain. Everyone in the restaurant was like a character out of a sitcom too edgy for the networks. Rich was oversensitive, especially when anyone touched his favorite knife, and he often stormed out the back door muttering obscenities, taking his knife with him. The grizzled old man who washed dishes was an unrepentant satyr who talked about becoming a superhero named Super Cock. Erica often gave coffee and sandwiches to homeless people, and she worried over the fate of a prostitute who lived in an apartment behind Banyan's tiny parking lot. When the ladies from the Junior League drove up to the restaurant, they would sometimes see this woman bidding her johns farewell at her open door, wrapped in a raggedy kimono, her hair tousled in extravagant disarray. One day, when a man trotted off without paying, she chased him through the alley in her bare feet.

"Poor little ho," said Erica, shaking her head.

I graded my students' work at Banyan, and had written part of my third book there, and had navigated the emotions of transitioning from a newsroom to a university by going there every chance I got. It was no surprise, then, that I spent so much time perched at Banyan's counter as I grieved for my daughter.

On days when I felt like talking, Erica was ready to listen. She waited for me to bring it up, and as I told her what was happening, the babies dying around us and Junebug barely hanging on, she never talked about miracles or how all of this was God's will. When I pulled up photos of Junebug on my phone, she did not flinch.

Perpetual crisis defied easy summation. The endless setbacks, the slow-motion parade of fresh disasters—this was the new status quo of our lives. The complexity of it confounded some of our friends, who were committed to believing that everything was fine now that Junebug had survived the surgery.

"She's good now, right?" they would say. "When's she coming home?"

At first, Kelley and I had tried to explain about her lungs and her bowels and the swelling and the clot and the chylothorax. Our friends were patient and kind, but for many of them, the details from the hospital were too much. After ten minutes of listening politely, they would blink and look away and assure us that Junebug was a miracle. Maybe they just didn't know what else to say. Now when people we didn't know well asked about Junebug, we defaulted to vague.

"She's a fighter," we'd say. "But she has a long way to go."

We hated resorting to clichés, but they worked. We saw gratitude on these people's faces when they realized we were sparing them the twenty-minute forced march through our family's vale of tears. We had good friends and family who listened patiently whenever we called. I feared that we were asking too much of them, too, when each of them had kids who wanted to hear bedtime stories, dogs that needed walking so they wouldn't piss all over the laundry room, jobs where it was decidedly uncool to receive a call from your histrionic friend in the middle of every workday.

Even with Mike and Roy and our other closest friends, Kelley and I tried to pull back. We wanted them to dish with us like the old days, to recap whatever mindless show they'd watched on TV last night, to talk about whatever they wanted to talk about, instead of always worrying about us. Roy and I needed to grab the booth in Poets Corner and laugh when Erica served someone their risotto in a Plum bowl. We needed to revel in the glory of a ravishing woman strolling past, entering our field of vision just long enough to remind us that we were alive.

"The world is full of beauty," Roy often said when he saw someone particularly devastating, and he was right.

Kelley and I had to find some way back to all the things that we'd lost at the moment of our daughter's arrival. We needed to go to the Refinery, our favorite restaurant in Tampa, and order not one but two of their ridiculous desserts and talk about anything other than the hospital. We needed to reacquaint ourselves with what it was like to kiss. And when we returned to the NICU, we needed to appreciate another day with our little girl. Death could tag her whenever it wanted, yes. But death was coming for all of us, sooner or later. Death could take me or Kelley or Roy or Erica or anyone else, at any moment.

Kelley and I needed a dose of faith, not to believe that Junebug would live, but to recognize that she was alive right now. Even if she never made it out of that room, we had to find a way to show her the world's beauty and joy, the things that made sorrow bearable.

Our daughter was right in front of us. Her eyes were open, her ears could hear, she felt our fingertips on her skin. Her mind was a blank canvas, ready for new data, experiences, sensations.

Her moment was now.

The doctors whittled away at the list of threats.

An ophthalmologist had begun to examine her periodically

to see if the oxygen was damaging her retinas. Junebug hated his exams even more than she'd hated the insertion of the catheter, because the doctor held her eyes open with metal clips attached to her eyelids, as in *A Clockwork Orange*. After several exams, he informed us that our daughter was showing retinal damage at what he called stage two plus, and that this damage was exacerbated by the presence of "popcorn," small isolated tufts of neovascular tissue on the surface of her retinas. The popcorn was an ominous sign that the damage was worsening. The doctor said Juniper would soon need laser eye surgery and would probably end up at least partially blind.

"I'd rather she be blind than dead," Kelley said.

"Me, too."

Almost everything the doctors did came with a price, and pretending otherwise would only make things harder. The doctors still had no idea what the surgeon would find when she cut back into Juniper's abdomen. I kept staring at the incision, which wound across her belly like the Euphrates. The gaps where her drains had fallen out were not yet fully closed, and I saw something gray beneath.

"Are those her intestines?" I asked Dr. Walford when she stopped by one day to check her patient's progress.

She was kind enough not to laugh.

"No," she said, explaining that it was fibrin, a protein that forms chains of polymers to help the blood clot over a wound. "It's part of the body's healing process."

The surgeon had not seen Junebug in ten days, because she'd gotten married and been off on her honeymoon. When she saw her patient under the light, she was startled.

"Wow. She's grown."

Dr. Walford glanced my way.

"How's Mom doing?"

I paused. Should I be polite and say Kelley was fine? Or should I tell her the truth and say that she was up and down? Dr. Walford read all of it on my face. She nodded to say she understood. How many couples had she seen going through this? How many marriages had come apart here on Six South? Given that she was newly wed, would it be rude to ask?

"Day by day," she said, then took off her gloves and headed for another patient.

Not long after Dr. Walford's exam, poop made a surprise reappearance in our daughter's diapers. Her fistula had closed, all on its own. The perforations in her intestines had closed, all on their own. Her body had somehow managed to resume digestion, all on its own. No one was talking about short gut anymore, or the need for another surgery.

"Wait, wait," I said after Diane explained the good news. "Are you telling me her body healed itself?"

"Yep," she said, grinning. "Your daughter is amazing."

Next on the schedule was the battle against the chylothorax. Fluid was still pouring from her chest, and they had yet to figure out why. They were preparing to attack the problem by starting her on a drug called octreotide, but first, Dr. Germain pulled me aside to get my permission. He told me that there was almost nothing in the medical literature on the use of this drug with a micro-preemie. They had no idea if the octreotide would work, and they could not assure me with any confidence that the drug would not hurt my daughter in some way they could not predict.

I had come a long way since the day I'd wanted to punch this man. Now I appreciated his caution and directness. The delicate and slightly melancholy way he spoke — the modulated calm that had so enraged me at our first encounter—was not his way of patronizing me. According to Tracy and everyone else I asked, he was just a super-sweet guy. Sometimes, if one of his patients was on the edge, he worried so much that he couldn't sleep. The kindness of it made me want to hug him, but I didn't want to scare him.

"Do we have any other choice?" I asked.

He thought for a minute, his eyes never breaking contact with mine, before he answered.

"Not really."

Kelley

It was unsettling to think about what all this care was costing. Those thoughts led to hard questions about what Juniper's life, or anyone's life, is worth. One afternoon I stopped by the newspaper to take care of some paperwork. A friend gave me a hug and then asked me a difficult question, trusting that I knew she meant no harm.

"Don't take this the wrong way," she said, "but wouldn't it be better to vaccinate a million kids in Africa?"

A lot of people wondered the same thing, I knew. Health care was not strictly a personal issue. One way or another, we all shared the costs. If Tom and I had still been on the newspaper's insurance plan, we probably would have wrecked everyone's premiums. How does one long-shot baby justify so much expense when so many people go without insurance?

I could have debated with her for an hour. We can never know what an investment in a child's life will reap. We can't predict the serendipitous discoveries that come from audacious endeavors. If we don't deny health care to the very old, why would we deny it to the newly born?

My friend was smart, so I didn't want to spout off. The answer is complicated.

Babies born earlier than twenty-eight weeks gestation required an average of about $200,000 in medical care by age seven. Juniper had already exceeded that easily. The statements that arrived almost daily from our insurance company told part of the story. The neonatologists cost about $1,900 a day. A month in the NICU—presumably room, board, and nursing care—was billed at between $200,000 and $450,000. Then there were the costs for surgeries, lab work, and specialists. All together, Juniper's care cost more than $6,000 a day.

Neonatal intensive care for the sickest babies was the most expensive intervention in pediatrics. But that didn't mean it was a bad deal. Medicaid and insurance companies paid willingly, which made NICUs profit centers for many hospitals. The care of micro-preemies subsidized other services for other kids.

In the NICU, ninety cents of every dollar was spent on kids who survived. That proved true even for the tiniest babies. Part of the reason was that the sickest babies tended to die in the first few days, before their hospital tabs ran too high. By contrast, most of the dollars spent on the elderly went to patients who died without ever leaving the hospital—costly and desperate attempts to buy another week or month with surgery, radiation, dialysis, a tracheotomy, a ventilator. The NICU was a bargain compared with adult intensive care, because dollars spent there bought many more years of life.

So, would it be better to spend the money on a million kids in Africa?

Standing there with my friend, I didn't wade into the complexities. I just answered honestly and reflexively, like any desperate new mom.

"Better for who?"

Tom

I had come to love the yawning time just after dawn. When Tracy slipped away to check on her other patients, I held Junebug's hand and read to her quietly with a tiny spider light clipped to the book, beaming a thin ray onto the page and allowing me to see her face turned toward mine. Her eyes always stared up at me with what looked like expectation.

By now the sun was blazing outside, the hospital's exterior melting in the liquid embrace of a subtropical summer, but my daughter's room stayed cool and dark. I reveled in that darkness. I thought of it as hers and mine, a velvet blanket that hid us from the world like an invisibility cloak, a den where we were hibernating together, both of us changing into someone new. A black star, stunning in its desolate beauty, drawing us into an orbit of quantum possibilities, ghost realities, an array of superpositions that were never fixed, where death could not pin us down.

Mary the cleaning lady came in every morning with her mop and saw me standing over the incubator, turning the pages of the book. The nod she gave humbled me every time.

"Keep going, Dad," she'd say. "Your little girl is listening."

We had finished book 1 of the *Harry Potter* series, thank

God, and were deep into book 2, with the flying car and the unjust imprisonment of Hagrid and the spiders and the giant snake flicking its tongue inside the subterranean Chamber of Secrets. Junebug always satted near a hundred when I came to the parts about Dobby, the character most like her. The truth was, she looked quite a bit like a house elf.

When she drifted off I would close the book and turn off the spider light and study her face beneath the tape and the tubes. Now that the swelling was finally going down, I could see the child she was becoming. It made me laugh, that face, the way she shifted so quickly from irritation to contentment to blissful confusion. Sometimes when Junebug was asleep I would silently thank J. K. Rowling for creating something of such enchantment, for giving my daughter the first story she had ever heard and making sure it was a good one. I was pretty sure Rowling would understand Junebug, because her books followed a child who did not know who he was, who endured losses and pain that might have crushed him, who longed for his parents to stand beside him and who triumphed over death again and again.

Now that we were in a private room, I felt free to play Junebug some music. I played her the Decemberists singing "June Hymn," because I'd sung it to her in the womb. I played her Stevie Wonder, because he'd been born a preemie, too, and because she always satted high for his soaring voice. I played her the Beatles and the Rolling Stones, Otis Redding and Aretha Franklin, Roy Orbison and Elvis, Bill Withers and Simon and Garfunkel and Wilco and Weezer. I played trashy songs that my sister Brooke and I had loved in the seventies: "Patches" and "Signs" and "Joy to the World." I played her the sound track from *Mary Poppins,* though neither Tracy nor Kelley could tolerate it when I played "Feed the Birds," about an old woman in London selling bags of bread crumbs so people could feed the pigeons that flocked on the steps outside St. Paul's Cathedral. Allegedly it had been Walt Disney's favorite song, but my wife and our nurse were having none of it.

"It just goes on and on," said Kelley.

"All that flapping of the wings," said Tracy. " 'Tuppence a bag, tuppence a bag.' "

"We've had it with tuppences."

Of course, I played loads of Springsteen: "Wild Billy's Circus Story," "Tenth Avenue Freeze-Out," "The Promised Land," "The River," Bruce's cover of Tom Waits's "Jersey Girl," the live version of "Racing in the Street," from one of the Meadowlands shows in the summer of 1981, with Roy Bittan's sweeping piano solo at the end. I told Junebug about the dozens of times I'd seen Springsteen in concert and how it always felt as though he were saying things already in my head that I could never put to words. I told her how I'd met Springsteen when I was still a college student, after a concert in South Bend. After the marathon show ended, my friends and I had stopped at a Big Boy restaurant south of town. When Springsteen and the E Street Band walked in a few minutes later, I worked up the courage to approach with my notebook and ask for an interview. Exhausted as Springsteen was, he patiently answered all of my questions and was polite enough not to comment on the fact that my hands were shaking. I told him how my friends and I endlessly debated a line from "Streets of Fire," about a voice calling his name in the darkness. Was the voice in front of Springsteen or behind him?

"You're thinkin' too hard, kid," he said, laughing.

Junebug, equally patient, listened to all my stories and kept satting high. I wanted her to understand why I had taken Nat and Sam to Springsteen shows since they were in elementary school, and why I was looking forward to the day when she could ride our shoulders in front of the stage and sing along to "Thunder Road."

Kelley introduced Junebug to Dylan, Al Green, John Prine, and Johnny Cash. One afternoon I walked in and she was holding our baby and singing "Folsom Prison Blues," telling Junebug that she had shot a man in Reno, just to watch him die. I didn't think it was possible to love someone as much as I loved my wife at that moment.

When her mother wasn't in the room, I told Junebug the story of how we'd met when Kelley was in high school and how if I'd tried to date her then I would have been arrested. I told her how we'd met again so many years later, and how we'd kissed and what a jerk I'd been, running from her for so long. I told her about her mom's dream about running me over with the car, and about my epiphany among the gargoyles, and how I'd crawled on my belly to win her back. When her mom walked down the aisle in her dress, I said, she'd looked so beautiful that I was sure I didn't deserve her.

After Junebug fell asleep, I remembered other parts of the story that weren't for a child's ears. The midnight drives that led me to that young woman waiting in the front window, smiling shyly. A first kiss that lasted nine hours. The look on her face in the triage room when she was covered in the half-digested blueberries, begging me not to let her die. All that blood. The night we heard Dr. Germain's statistics and sat up till dawn, trying to figure out what was right for our little girl. In the delivery room,

Kelley looking at them wheeling the baby away, then looking at me.

Go.

Across the room my daughter stirred, and I picked up *The Chamber of Secrets* again. We were ready for the last chapter, where Dobby is finally set free after a lifetime of servitude. We finished book 2 that night, and the next morning we dove into book 3, Junebug satting high with every page. She had just been listening to the first chapter when they opened the incubator to change her diaper. Ana Maria, the physical therapist, was massaging Junebug's shoulder when she turned and motioned me closer. Junebug had heard my voice and was looking in my direction, and when I leaned in, I could hear the slightest hint of a scratchy sound coming out of her mouth, past her vent.

Ana Maria smiled.

"She's talking to you."

Day of Life 49.

A lazy Monday afternoon, no new crises, nothing remarkable. Junebug's chest tubes had leaked fluid, so Tracy needed to change her bedding. She asked me to lift the baby slightly out of the way while she stripped the sheets. To make it work, I had to bend at a weird angle and hold the ventilator tube.

Tracy was bustling back and forth, and then she didn't get the bedding the way she wanted, so she had to start over. More bustling, and I heard her pushing one of the tall chairs up behind me.

"For your back," she said, then disappeared.

Suddenly I realized that I was holding my daughter in my

arms, not just lifting her like a package. I pulled her close and looked down at her, and she looked up in my direction.

I cleared my throat and started to sing. My voice was rough, but Junebug didn't seem to mind. Only one song would do, and she had heard it many times before. The screen door was slamming, and Mary's dress was waving in the night.

Kelley

I was in the car when Tracy texted me the photo, from Tom's phone.

Juniper was wrapped in a green blanket with her little hands sticking out by her face, like she was either waving or pontificating. She looked like a shrunken, bundled Pope. Tom looked just as bleary and exhausted as any new dad holding his daughter for the first time. She rested on one of his forearms. He'd been waiting to hold her for seven weeks.

I'd been waiting to see him hold our daughter for five years, if you count from when we started trying to have a baby. Or nine years, if you count from that first forever-long kiss. Or my whole life, if you want to know the truth.

I jerked the car in the direction of the hospital. I got there in plenty of time. She was content, and there was no need to rush. I got to wrap my arms around his shoulders and take a family selfie and listen to him serenade our daughter with "Blue Bayou." The gurgling of the chest tubes and the whooshing of the ventilator didn't matter. Tom was singing about his worried mind and his lonely heart and how he was saving nickels and dimes and working past exhaustion, all so he could take his baby home and hold her tight as they watched the silver moon rising.

Maybe I'll be happy then on Blue Bayou

Happy is such a shallow word. It can't contain what I felt, being in that room. My husband was beautiful, with his dirty T-shirt and his unwashed hair, his voice cracking and faltering. I wanted to *inhabit* him.

To say that my daughter looked like a doll would sound clichéd. People who describe their daughters as looking like dolls do not actually have doll-size daughters. She was a magical, live-action doll, who wiggled and waved.

She blinked up at him with something like skepticism, then awe, then annoyance, then contentment, then bemusement.

I didn't feel anything as slight as happiness. I didn't feel euphoria or joy or any emotion so fleeting or pure. I felt complete. I felt full. I felt okay. We were okay, right now. I would have this moment forever, no matter what came next.

No one could tell us if or when it was going to be permanently okay. Seeing Tom hold our daughter was like emerging momentarily from the tunnel, just before plunging back into the dark. Everyone told us we were on a roller coaster or a journey, metaphors that made me gag. If it was a roller coaster, it was a rickety one with no brakes.

Desperate for something to focus me, I bought a whiteboard and stuck it to the wall in her room.

> *To Do*
> ✓ *Survive birth*
>   *Breathe (ongoing)*
> ✓ *Heal tummy*
> ✓ *Win over Tracy*
> ✓ *1000 grams*
>   *2000 grams*
>   *Off the ventilator*

Off oxygen
Lose chest tubes
Dissolve blood clot
Learn to eat
Acquire pony

Tom considered the list and then added:

Conquer space and time

I also posted a Freak-Out Level Indicator, color-coded, because I was never sure when my level of alarm matched the doctors'. Most days were yellow—caution. To get to green, she had to stop setting off the alarms.

Slowly the doctors started reintroducing tiny amounts of milk into the tube that snaked into Juniper's belly. Nothing calamitous happened. Breast milk was tricky because it contained long-chain triglycerides, exactly the type of fat that caused her chest to spurt fluid. I would have understood if the doctors had just said that given the circumstances Similac would do, but the benefits were worth the trouble. The milk contained leukocytes, antibodies, enzymes, and hormones that couldn't be replicated in formula.

The lactation consultants put the milk in a centrifuge and spun it, then scraped off the fat, turning whole milk into skim. They encouraged me to perform a series of science experiments at home. I lined up the little bottles on my kitchen counter, and using borrowed hospital supplies, I ran tubing into the bottles. I'd chill the milk, trying to get the fat to congeal at the surface, horrifying my visiting stepsons when they opened the fridge looking for a Frappuccino.

I brought in various samples to be tested for fat content. Morning milk, night milk, foremilk, hindmilk. Moms will know what I'm talking about here, and dads won't want to know.

The lactation consultants seemed excited about the project. They spent most of their time preaching the Gospel of the Liquid Gold to reluctant or fed-up moms. It was noble work. I imagined their days were filled with nipples—cracked, bleeding, plugged, inverted, yeasty—and with weeping mothers and angry babies. One of the lactation consultants carried a stuffed monkey in order to demonstrate proper technique. Every time I saw her in the halls with that giant purple fur baby clinging to her neck, I hid.

"The lactation consultants were looking for you again," Tracy said one day.

"The one with the monkey?"

"Not the monkey one, no."

If the issues could be overly technical, the progress could also be mind-numbingly incremental. The baby was so sensitive to change that the most gradual weaning of a drug could be too much for her. Rather than lower a dose, they had to wait for her to outgrow it. But once in a while, to balance the precipitous calamities we'd endured, something wonderful would happen, out of nowhere.

On Juniper's fifty-ninth day, with little fanfare or warning, Tracy took her off the ventilator. Just for a second, I saw my daughter's whole face.

The tube came out, and Tracy propped her up in her hand long enough for me to take a picture. I could see that she looked like Jennifer, because Jennifer has a cute nose and a wide upper lip, and there they were, in miniature. Juniper's lip was red from the tape that had stuck to it since birth. She had a deep wrinkle in the left corner of her mouth, where it had permanently creased. Tracy put a cannula in her nose, which made her look even more like an old man on oxygen. She still had a thin tube running into her mouth and into her stomach, but now she could close her mouth. She could suck a pacifier, which was smaller than a pencil eraser. And she could cry.

At first, her voice was tiny and hoarse. She mewled. It quickly strengthened, to a squeak like a rusty door hinge.

For two months we had watched her writhe mutely. Now her cries were staggering. They were a testament not only to her strength, but to the technology that had propped open her flimsy lungs until they could function. Juniper's lungs were scarred, maybe permanently. But her scratchy cry was a marvel. It was a triumph. It was an announcement.

People clash over the question of when life begins and when a fetus becomes a human being with its own standing and stake in the world. I never saw Juniper as pre-human. Even on her first perilous day, four months before she was supposed to be born, I witnessed her individuality and her will. But there was something sacred about watching her take shape in the incubator as she would have in my womb. When the ventilator came out, I saw that from under so much hardware, a little girl had emerged.

She had opinions. She felt pain, irritation, discontent, outrage. For the first time, she had a voice.

If she'd been born that day, in June, she would still have been two months premature. But she looked like a baby now, only smaller. She looked like one of those itty-bitty baby dolls toddlers drag around by the leg.

Now that Juniper was freed from the ventilator, Tracy grew bolder in her accessorizing. We'd heard that she had once dressed a baby in a blue top hat, bow tie, cummerbund, and cuffs and tucked a tiny dollar bill into his diaper. A Chippen-preemie. She'd created a UPS driver, a nurse, a boxer in a boxing-ring incubator, and Rudolph the Red-Nosed Reindeer. She'd wrapped one in gauze like a mummy in a haunted incu-bator crawling with plastic spiders. The preemies always cooperated.

One summer afternoon, we dressed Juniper in a pink polka-dot bikini made for a doll. She had a tiny beach ball and a tote bag slung over one shoulder.

Jennifer and her kids were at the beach that day. I texted them a photo.

Joining you in spirit, I typed.

In mid-June, during slow periods when Juniper was sleeping, Tracy began work on her greatest stunt. She took a piece of dark felt from her purse and cut it into two pieces shaped like a *T*. She hand-stitched it up both sides, and put a slit in the front for the wires. She was careful to hide the tiny outfit when anyone was around, so she wouldn't ruin the surprise. She locked it in a drawer, bagged and labeled so the other nurses wouldn't throw it out.

Tracy was starting to see Juniper react to things that could not be measured, prescribed, or ordered on rounds. She was not sentimental, but she was starting to believe the risk she'd taken by letting herself get attached had been worth it.

When I watched Tracy lean close to Juniper and whisper, or stroke her head with a fingertip, or dress her up like a Chihua-hua at a dinner party, I knew she didn't just take care of our baby. She loved her.

Together one afternoon, Tracy and I broke the sticks off cotton swabs to make a tiny broomstick. Tracy had a superstition against dressing babies in eyeglasses, eye patches, fake casts, peg legs, or anything that might portend a future disability. But this costume demanded round eyeglasses and a lightning-bolt scar.

She cut out the glasses from a black hospital mask and drew the scar on a piece of clear tape. When the time came, just before Tom visited one afternoon, she slipped Juniper into the T-shaped robe and stuck the scar on her forehead.

Happy Father's Day. From Harry Potter.

Tom

We were getting too comfortable, starting to relax, tempting the patience of the gods.

One morning late that June, we were ranging deep inside book 3, Junebug and I. We had finished reading about Sirius Black's escape from the Dementors at Azkaban. The room around us was swimming in that beautiful darkness, and the tiny beam of my spider light was shining on the pages resting on the incubator. Junebug was looking up at me, listening and watching, and on the monitor her aqua sat number pinged at one hundred. We were just about to read the part where Scabbers, Ron's pathetic rat, is revealed to be Wormtail, Voldemort's henchman, when suddenly the alarms went off, and Junebug began to desat rapidly, past ninety, past eighty...

I closed the book and shook her shoulder to remind her to breathe. But her heart rate had slowed, and the sat number on the monitor kept plunging. It was like watching her free-fall from the top of a skyscraper.

When Tracy heard the alarms, she came running with a respiratory team. I backed away and gave them room as they flipped on the lights and popped the top of her box and sat her up and put a plastic bag over her mouth and nose and began squeezing the bag, pushing oxygen into her lungs. They were pounding her back and calling out to her. They were begging.

Down past sixty, past fifty...

Junebug's eyes were open, and they were scanning the nurses' faces. Was she looking for me? Her skin, pink only a minute or so before, was blue now and draining toward gray.

Forty...

"Come on, Juniper!" said Tracy. "Breathe! Come on!"

Thirty...

I was holding the book and holding my breath. I wanted them to turn out the lights and let us rewind the tape, so that we could return to the darkness and the refuge of the story.

Twenty...

"Breathe, Junebug! Breathe!"

She was close to zero when she came back to us. The aqua number began to rise, and her heart rate broke into jagged beats, and her skin shifted back toward pink. Tracy stayed close, fidgeting and worrying and rearranging. When she relaxed, I went back to the incubator and looked down at my daughter, reminding myself that she was still here.

Now that Junebug was off the ventilator, breathing more on her own, her body was struggling to keep up. She was repeatedly suffering episodes of apnea, where her lungs went still, as well as episodes of bradycardia, where her heart slowed. Sometimes these crises struck ten times a day.

That same morning, as Junebug and I plowed through the final chapters of book 3, Dr. Raj stopped by at rounds and tried to figure out why she'd plunged so dramatically a couple of hours before. Chest X-rays had been ordered, and now he was calling up the results on his computer. He pointed to a large white blob on her right side.

"She's whited out," he said.

Either she had suffered a collapsed lung that morning, Raj said, or more fluid was pooling around the lung and applying pressure, making it harder for her to breathe.

The doctor was talking about what to do next when the monitor alarms cut him off. Once again, Junebug's heart rate and sat level were dropping. Tracy was sitting her up. They were bagging her again.

"She's bradying right now," said Tracy.

"Is she apneic?" asked Raj.

"She's apneic."

Tracy was still holding the bag over Junebug's face, watching her sat level climb back into the nineties.

"Juniper," she said, "what's up with you?"

Despite the progress we'd been making, we knew we could still lose her. The blood clot was shrinking but still clung inside her heart. Her lungs still needed supplemental oxygen, especially with the fluid in her chest. In the course of a single day, she would soar, plummet, soar again. The oxygen dance, the nurses called it, and until she grew stronger, the dance would not stop.

That day, Junebug and I finished book 3, and I could tell that she was happy—or whatever a neonatologist would call it—when Harry and Hermione used the time-turner to save Buckbeak from the executioner's blade and then climbed onto the hippogriff's back and flew into the night to save Sirius from the Dementors. The daring rescue had always been one of my favorite moments in the series, and I was sure that my daughter could hear it in my voice.

In the days that followed, we galloped through book 4. In

that darkness I told her stories about her mother and how she loved horses as a little girl and how she used to ride one to a Baskin-Robbins for ice cream on hot summer days. I told her stories from her brothers' childhoods, Nat's worship of Isaac Newton, Sam's worship of any baker who delivered doughnuts into his life. One day, when Kelley and I were sitting together with her, we shared a short list of life rules that the boys and I had compiled when they were growing up.

1. Never hit a cop.
2. Never call your mother a drunken whore, as one of Sam's friends had once done, thinking she was being funny.
3. Never piss off Bob Dylan, because he will write a song about you, and the song will be so good that his scorn will live forever.

To prove it, I let her listen to "Positively Fourth Street."

When I grew tired of reading and ran out of embarrassing anecdotes, I recited the first twenty pages or so of *A Christmas Carol*. The holidays were months away, but I didn't care. I loved the audio recording of the book performed by Patrick Stewart, and I played it relentlessly every year from Thanksgiving on. I'd memorized long passages and could mimic the various accents and voices that Stewart had invented. Every time I started, it drove Kelley and the boys crazy.

" 'Marley was dead: to begin with…' " I would say.

Sam would roll his eyes and chime in. " 'There is no doubt whatever about that.' "

Then Nat: " 'Marley was as dead as a doornail.' "

Junebug didn't protest when I regaled her with Dickens. She didn't know it was summer.

"'Oh! But he was a tight-fisted hand at the grindstone, Scrooge! a squeezing, wrenching, grasping, scraping, clutching, covetous old sinner...'"

Tracy would give me a look, but I kept going.

"'Hard and sharp as flint, from which no steel had ever struck generous fire; secret, and self-contained, and solitary as an oyster.'"

I wished I'd written those lines. My immersion in the story had made me believe that Dickens had identified with Scrooge and had written the story to remind himself what can happen to a man ruled by fear—a moral that held particular power for me. I had convinced myself that Tiny Tim had been a preemie and that his body had never recovered. That accounted for why his father, Bob Cratchit, was so protective. I heard Patrick Stewart rendering Tim's ragged voice at the dinner table, calling out a feeble "Hurrah," and I saw my daughter sitting among the Cratchits, clamoring for her portion of the Christmas goose.

One day when Tracy put a long dark wig on her, it reminded me of the singer Melanie. I was inspired to serenade my daughter with a falsetto "I've got a brand-new pair of roller skates," which made Tracy laugh. Somewhere in that long summer, I came up with a modified version of "The Hokey Pokey."

You put your ventilator in, you put your ventilator out
You put your ventilator in, and you shake it all about.
You do the Preemie Pokey and you turn yourself
*   around.*
That's what it's all about.

When nothing else calmed Junebug down, "The Preemie Pokey"
worked.

You put your Broviac in, you put your Broviac out…

Almost every night, I played my daughter "My Sweet Lord."
George Harrison's voice had followed me since the first time I'd
heard the song, back in sixth grade. I didn't care if he was
talking about Hare Krishnas or if the chanting at the end made
any sense. For me, "My Sweet Lord" was one of the most tran-
scendent pieces of music anyone had ever created. Harrison had
written a song about wanting to see the face of God, and he had
dared to release it into the predatory marketplace of commercial
radio. It was as though Jesus had delivered a sermon while
standing among the money changers who had invaded the temple. The naked yearning in Harrison's voice was almost painful
to contemplate. For so much of his life, he had wanted to be
with God. And now he was.

Sitting for so long in that darkness, I thought a great deal
about God and what that word meant to me. I had no use for
the version the nuns had tried to sell me during catechism.
The bearded sage, condemning people to eternal fire? He
sounded like an embittered old man, boarded up in his house
at the end of the road, living out of coffee cans, spitting out
curses at all those who had disagreed with him. As best I
could tell, God was not an entity at all, but a force gathered
inside anything and everything that had meaning. When I
saw my daughter's hand, gripping her mother's finger, I believed
in God. When I sang to my child the sweet and raucous songs
that had shaped me, that was my way of praying. When I

escaped with Junebug inside a children's book where her brothers' younger selves lived on, we were all taking communion
together.

"The world consists of the tension between order and
chaos," a mathematician had once told the *New York Times*.
Every hour of every day, the forces of randomness exerted their
claim. Tornadoes descended from above and tore through nursing homes. Cancer cells blossomed inside otherwise healthy
children. Black holes devoured galaxies. Dark energy, invisible
to NASA's telescopes and beyond scientists' comprehension,
pushed the accelerator on the expansion of the universe, sending
us farther into the void.

In the darkness of Junebug's room and in the light of everything beyond, stories were my best defense against randomness.
If the world was defined by the tension between order and
chaos, then our lives unfolded in perpetual countercurrents of
meaning and meaninglessness. I saw it whenever I walked into
the NICU, where the alarms were constantly sounding. The
songs we sang, the books we read—all of them helped keep our
family afloat. They calmed us, inspired us, helped us hang on
through the long months of not knowing how our daughter's
story would end. Every time we opened to another page of
Harry Potter, the story transported us into other lives and other
experiences that echoed our own. They helped the three of us
imagine a future after the hospital. They told our daughter she
was not alone.

Junebug's favorite song was "Waitin' On a Sunny Day." I had
once read an interview with Springsteen where he admitted that
"Sunny Day" was not his most elegant piece of work. But the
song did what he designed it to do, which was to make people

rise up out of their seats, and it had a breathless propulsion that I had always loved. When we played it for our daughter, she always satted high, which made sense, because she had never felt the sun on her skin.

The song was about a man who longed for someone he loved to come home. It described the inevitability of hard times and the power of love to overcome those obstacles. The images contained inside the lyrics were a catalog of things our daughter had never experienced: Rain falling onto her skin. A dog barking in the distance, the call of an ice cream truck on an empty street. The ticking of a clock on the wall. Night, giving way to morning.

Springsteen did not know my little girl, but he had sent this song out into the ether and it had found its way into this permanent darkness where she lived, into this box where she was confined, and when I hit "play" on my phone, she could hear his voice—a voice that had been singing in my ear for most of my sorry life, guiding me forward. He was creating a world of new sensations for my daughter, and every time I played it for her, he promised her what I did not dare to promise. Someday we would find a way out of this place.

Don't worry, we're gonna find a way
Don't worry, we're gonna find a way

I was in the room one day late that June when Kelley came running in. Clarence Clemons, Springsteen's legendary sax player, had suffered a stroke a few days before, and now he was gone at age sixty-nine. Kelley and I told Junebug we were sorry she would never get to see Clarence riding that long, hypnotic solo in "Jungleland." That day I played her the song with Kelley leaning against my shoulder. We didn't sing along, because we wanted our daughter to hear every note. We wanted her to feel the music wrapping around us and weaving through us, the way it filled us and broke us, then put us back together and drifted away.

Through all of it, Junebug held very still, her dark eyes watching.

Kelley

During the months Juniper spent in the NICU, the children of a half-dozen of our friends came through the hospital—for scoliosis surgery, a birth, a ballooned appendix, a cardiac checkup. One day, by the sign-in desk, we introduced ourselves to the daughter of our accountant. Danielle and her husband were still shaken by the news that their son, born with Down syndrome, needed surgery. Their faces were clouded with exhaustion and fear, but something else, too. Joy.

"We just can't wait to take him home and love him," Danielle's husband said.

I visited baby Jack in his room, which was papered in hand-drawn welcome posters and filled with books.

"Can you hold Juniper yet?" Danielle asked.

"I haven't for a long time," I said.

Danielle scooped up Jack and plopped him in my arms, just like that. I couldn't remember the last time I'd held a full-size baby. Jack was all soft cheeks and soft breath and soft hair. He was so much rounder than Juniper, with his pudgy baby arms and those sweet wrinkles in his neck. His parents hadn't known about the Down syndrome until he was born. They said it didn't matter. I envied them for that. He was exquisite, but in his extra chromosome, I saw a parallel to our worst fears.

Doctors had told us Juniper would probably be disabled. We'd considered letting her die rather than face the odds. Why had we struggled so much, when Jack's parents seemed so content?

Many of us have grown comfortable with kids with Down syndrome. But not so long ago, things were different. In 1982, the parents of an Indiana baby with Down syndrome declined an esophageal surgery that would have saved his life. The case got national attention, and the surgeon general argued that it was child abuse to withhold treatment from a baby because of a mental handicap. The Baby Doe case forced doctors, hospitals, and parents to reevaluate how they weighed quality of life.

Thirty years later, parents still struggled with a diagnosis of Down syndrome, and most aborted their babies after prenatal testing. But once a child was born with the condition, there was a consensus to treat them. Kids with Down syndrome were in Target ads. There was even one on *Glee*.

So why, then, did the prospect of disability in the earliest preemies like Juniper feel like a death sentence? Some micro-preemies would grow up with profound disadvantages, as would Jack, but others would be indistinguishable from kids born full term. Maybe it was easier to confront a familiar condition like Down syndrome than a buffet of unknowns.

Jack's mom was putting no limits on his potential. She read to him in the NICU from the day he was born. "We have no idea what he will be capable of," she told me. And why not? I'd seen adults with Down syndrome in wedding dresses and in caps and gowns, despite our society's short history of giving them a fair chance. What could a kid like Jack do with a mom like Danielle?

I wished for a little of the certainty I saw in her. For me, every day in the NICU had been a lesson in humility and patience and accepting risk. Danielle inspired me to ask a new question: What could a kid like Juniper do with a mom like me?

I'd seen how she responded to my voice. I'd discovered that I had an intuition about her that even Tom didn't have. I took home her blankets every night and washed them, burying my face in them before tossing them in the machine. I fed her from my body. Being her mom wasn't something I might get to do someday. It was something I did now, every day. Tom had been right. It was mostly about showing up. I had learned how to show up.

I still wanted her to ride horses and run marathons and win the spelling bee. But I read something that helped me maintain perspective. In an essay, a Canadian neonatologist named Annie Janvier recalled a young family whose premature baby had suffered a debilitating brain bleed. Debating whether to take the baby off life support, the boy's father asked the doctor a series of befuddling questions.

"Will I love him even though he's disabled?"

Of course.

"Will he love us?"

Just as any other child loves his parents.

"Will he be able to have sex?"

That one made the doctor pause. There was no physical reason he couldn't.

"Will he be able to make pizza?"

It turned out the couple worked together in the family pizza shop. They had a simple life. They loved each other, they made pizza, they watched movies, they had sex. They were happy. They knew that if their son could do those things, he could be happy too.

So why did I want Juniper to have not just a driver's license, but a pilot's license; not just a love of music, but front-row seats for Springsteen; not just an education, but a graduate degree in a fulfilling and creative discipline, hopefully leading swiftly to a lucrative and rewarding career that afforded her the opportunity to both change the world and spend abundant time with my grandchildren, all seven of them?

Tom and I wanted the whole world for her, but it would have to be the world she sought, not one we designed. We knew even less about her potential than Danielle knew about Jack's. If she wore glasses, or developed asthma, or limped or lugged around an oxygen tank, would she be less amazing? If she worked in a pizza shop, would she be less loved?

"She's the strongest person I have ever known," Tom said. "She doesn't have to prove anything to me, ever."

When I got back to her room, I held her hand, noticing that it was a normal color now, neither translucent nor angry red nor poisoned brown. Just a tiny baby hand, between my forefinger and thumb. I promised her that whatever her life became, it would be better for having been our kid.

Tracy left the top up on the incubator all the time now, giving Juniper's body time to learn to regulate its own temperature. Since I couldn't hold her, I would lower the sides of her incubator and lay my head next to her in the bed. We would stare at each other. We'd take selfies. She would sleep, and I'd close my eyes and pretend we were home.

At the end of June, an ultrasound showed that the clot in her heart had finally dissolved. After a few weeks of octreotide, the fluid pouring out of her body slowed and then stopped. The nurses clamped the chest tubes, then, mercifully, took them out.

She was nearing three pounds. Her features continued to plump and to soften. She was a distinct species from the fat babies in the regular nursery on the third floor. She could do a push-up and gaze all around the room. She had a wise look. She was stronger than any newborn, and her due date was still more than a month away.

Ana Maria said it was because she'd been doing calisthenics since she was born, constantly testing her muscles against the hard shell of the incubator. Juniper did other things newborns couldn't, too. She tracked us with her eyes, turning her head to follow us. She responded when we spoke to her. She smiled at us. She cried when we had to leave.

I don't care what the books say about newborn babies and smiles. That it's just gas, that it's a reflex. Whatever it is, I have video of it, and no journal article will convince me that what was happening in that time was anything other than a baby and a mother falling crazy in love, making stupid faces at each other all day long. In the video, it is July 12, and Juniper has just turned three months old. She's wearing the Aretha Franklin inauguration hat and lying on her zebra blanket. I tell her happy birthday, and she smiles. I kiss her on top of her head, and she smiles again.

"What do you want to do for your birthday?" I say. "Do you want some cuddles? Do you want some songs? Do you want to read a story? How about the one about Eeyore and the balloons, the one where he gets three presents?"

Her eyes wrinkle and she beams.

"Say hi to Daddy," I tell her.

She frowns. She never likes to perform on command.

Now that the chest tubes were out, we could hold her. As long as she was stable, we didn't even ask permission. We learned to gather up all the wires and tubes, which still dangled from her nose, mouth, hands, and feet, scoop her up, wrap her in a blanket, and rock her in the big recliner in the corner. She was no bigger than a sub sandwich.

She still stopped breathing. It happened sometimes when we were alone with her in the room—she'd just forget, turn gray, fall limp. Tom and I became experts at rubbing her back, prodding her to rejoin us in the here and now.

"Come on, Junebug," I'd say to her. *"Breathe."*

When she came to, she always looked startled, as if she wondered where she had been. I'd realize then that I'd been holding my breath, and release it with a rush. I would remind her that breathing was a thing she'd have to keep doing every day forever. When we describe something as effortless, we say it's "like breathing." But for her, it wasn't automatic, because the respiratory control center at the base of her brain was still developing. I thought about what a failure I'd been at yoga. Breathing consciously made me feel like I was going to have a panic attack. I couldn't imagine how it must have felt to be so small and have to pay such attention to the rise and fall of every breath.

"It'll get easier," I told her.

One day, the nurses rolled a crib into the room, and we rushed out to buy a baby mobile. I got one of those black-and-white modern-looking ones and realized within two days that it was made for moms, not babies, so back it went to the store. We got the plastic kind that spun and played music and cast constellations across the ceiling, and she watched it, enthralled, every moment that she was awake. Tracy brought a baby swing into the room and propped her in it, wires and all.

Ana Maria kept working with her, showing us how to relax her with our voices and hands. She taught me that in the incubator, babies lie too flat, too soon, which makes them tense and restricts their breathing. When their arms fall to the side they feel insecure, like they're floating. Ana Maria showed us how to tuck Juniper's knees under her, move her hands to her face, and prop her in pillows to hold her body in a nice round curl like a snail. Juniper loved Ana Maria. *She gets me,* I imagined her saying, as she melted into sleep.

Sam was home that whole summer. He came every day, holding and rocking her and entertaining her with embarrassing stories about their father.

The boys' mother, Linda, visited repeatedly, cooing at the baby.

"This is Nat's and Sam's little sister," she told us. "I'd like to get to know her if you'll allow it."

Mike finally got to hold her, too. When he lifted her for the first time, his eyes widened and he looked at me. "Oh my God," he said. "She's going to be fine."

By early July, her chart looked like this:

> *To Do*
> ✓ *Survive birth*
>   *Breathe (ongoing)*
> ✓ *Heal tummy*
> ✓ *Win over Tracy*
> ✓ *1000 grams*
>   *2000 grams*
> ✓ *Off the ventilator*
>   *Off oxygen*
> ✓ *Lose chest tubes*
> ✓ *Dissolve blood clot*
>   *Learn to eat*
>   *Acquire pony*
>   *Conquer space and time*

For a few weeks, she wore a CPAP oxygen mask attached to a little hat with a plastic cone that covered her nose. It was pretty much the same kind of elephantine apparatus that people who snore wear at night to prolong their marriages. On July Fourth weekend, the nurse lifted it off her face for a minute, and I saw that deep grooves had formed from the straps that held it on, making her look like the littlest lumpy-headed Munster. "Is this permanent?" I asked, and the nurse just chuckled. For five minutes, maybe ten, I rubbed Juniper's face and her tiny bobble-head in my hands, trying to restore her color, and she let her head just roll around, blissed out.

Diane came in.

"Did you see she's on full feeds?" she asked.

I looked over at the metal pole, which had once been so heavily laden and now grew lighter by the day. The bag of clear liquid nutrition was gone. Juniper had spent all seventy of her days on that stuff, which should have rotted her liver. Now she was getting fortified breast milk, seven milliliters per hour, through a tube.

Soon Diane would write an order to add vitamins and iron and to slowly reduce the octreotide.

"You might want to buy a car seat," she said. "She doesn't have too much left to accomplish here."

I'd waited months—no, years—for a reason to buy a car seat. Now, as Juniper's due date approached, Diane offered the first suggestion that she might leave the hospital. I felt a wave of euphoria, but it dissolved into nerves. All the rest of that day, Tom and I were a gloomy mess. Shaking and sometimes crying. Descending into silences.

"What is wrong with me?" Tom asked.

We took that night off from the NICU. We grabbed the dog,

Muppet, and her beloved tennis ball and headed to her favorite spot on earth, Fort De Soto beach, part of a glorious string of tiny islands off the southern tip of the Pinellas County peninsula.

It was a weeknight in July. Australian pines rose tall out of the sand next to the mangroves and sea oats. Bicyclists and Rollerbladers glided past the old fort and the campgrounds and kayak rentals. The dog beach was about halfway down, a little plot of sand just slightly less pure than the white powder of the more celebrated shorelines. We had it nearly to ourselves. We walked to the far end and flung the ball as Muppet tore after it. The wind was strong, and the waves were wrestling and racing each other to the shore. Muppet was all ears and tail and dancing feet.

Watching Muppet race down the beach and back, and down and back, I realized why we'd come undone. For months, we had coped by measuring time in minutes and hours. We had never looked ahead. We'd never dealt with the colossal risk of expectation. Now the sand was shifting. The hopes we had strangled for so long overwhelmed us.

Tom wrapped his arms around me. The dog ran down the beach and back.

PART FIVE

Sky

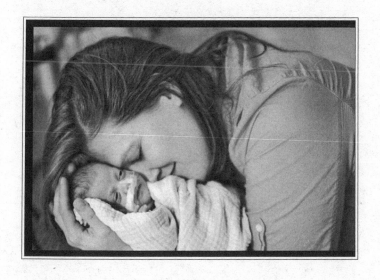

Kelley

August 3 arrived. My due date.

The date had been seared into my cortex for nearly a year, and reaching it felt like a milestone. But instead of a fat, red-faced newborn, I had a sick and hospitalized four-month-old. Tom was out of town. I didn't know how to feel.

From now forward, Juniper would have two ages: a real age and an adjusted age. Her birthday had been 113 days ago, but developmentally she was at day one.

Our nurse that day, Carol Tiffany, could read the mix of emotions on my face. I imagined she'd seen the look a thousand times before. She sent a patient-care assistant named Brooke to Labor and Delivery to fetch a rolling bassinet. Then Brooke and I stripped Juniper to her birthday suit and wrapped her in one of those blankets with the pink and blue footprints—the blanket you see in every Facebook photo of a new baby. We put a newborn hat on her head, and it fit. We weighed her: 4 pounds 10 ounces. We took handprints and footprints. Diane signed a ceremonial birth certificate and Brooke put a sign on Juniper's crib: HAPPY DUE DATE TO ME!

I tried to imagine what it would have been like if I'd given birth to her that day, having known nothing of the past four months, having never seen her as a twiggy one-pounder. I would have given anything to spare her the pain and to give her body that time in the womb to grow as it should, to have a nurse lay her on my sweaty chest, to see Tom fumbling the camera with tears on his face, to hear her piercing, healthy, room-rattling wail. But she and I would never have that moment. We were fundamentally different people now, forever.

We had been stuck in this Neverland between the womb and the world. It had transformed us. I had come to know her in a way that few mothers could ever know their children. I'd seen who she was at her raw core. I'd seen her as a nub, a sprouted seed. I'd witnessed her ferocity and her resolve. I'd watched her shape-shift. I'd watched her wake up.

Brooke and I stood now over her crib. Juniper could easily push herself up on her forearms and turn her head and survey the world as she knew it. She scanned the room and smiled.

I told Brooke about all the times I'd worried she would die. Brooke nodded. Part of her job, it turned out, was helping parents who have lost a baby. She would make handprints and footprints for those parents and present them with a hand-painted box. Volunteers made the boxes, she said. Inside was a little outfit, a lock of hair, some photos. They kept a supply of these boxes in a closet. Brooke called it the Dead Baby Closet.

"There were a few times they told me to get a box ready for Juniper, just in case."

When the blood drained out of my face, I tried not to let Brooke see me sway. I didn't mind learning these morsels of hard truth. It felt good to be trusted with our own reality.

A few days later, Juniper hit five pounds. I photographed her in her incubator next to a sack of sugar. Dr. Germain was on rounds that morning. Juniper wore a green hat with a purple double pompom. Dr. Germain looked smitten and proud. Someone called her a miracle.

Juniper was back to regular milk now. No more spinning off the fat. All that remained between her and freedom was to learn to eat from a bottle, to go several days without an episode of apnea, and, hopefully, to get off all the oxygen.

"She's officially almost boring," Dr. Germain said.

A day or two later, I stopped at the drugstore on the way to the hospital and picked up a stack of photos I'd had printed. I stood at the counter and flipped through them—from April to May to June to July—watching her evolve like a character in a jerky stop-motion movie. The early photos were still hard to look at. I wanted to post them in her hospital room so that everyone who flowed through her room every day could see in an instant how far she had come.

I planned to meet our friend Cherie at the NICU. When I arrived, a respiratory therapist was fiddling with the tube in Juniper's nose, and Juniper's oxygen was at 40 percent. It hadn't been that high in a long time.

"They just had rounds," he said. "You missed them by ten minutes."

The nurse hadn't mentioned any problems when I'd called that morning. Juniper was sleeping, wearing yellow duck pajamas with snaps up the leg and a matching hat. The nurse popped in and said the doctors had ordered an X-ray, but the results weren't in.

X-ray?

We didn't want to wake up Juniper, so Cherie and I went to lunch downtown. We talked about work, our colleagues, the anxiety in the newspaper business. By the time we left, I was desperate to get back to the NICU. I felt sure something was wrong.

When we returned, an ultrasound machine stood in the room, big as a dishwasher. The nurse seemed surprised to see it.

"When was that ordered?" she asked the tech.

"Just a bit ago. Stat."

I made eye contact with the nurse. "Will you please go find out what the hell is going on?" I asked.

No need. Dr. Stromquist walked in. The room was busy in a way I hadn't seen in weeks.

The X-ray showed more than an ounce of fluid on one side of Juniper's chest. The chylothorax had come back. Dr. Stromquist would draw out the fluid with a needle, and we were going to have to start spinning the fat off the milk again.

Cherie and I had to step out for the procedure, and when we came back fifteen minutes later, Juniper's room was full of people. She'd stopped breathing and her heart had stalled. Dr. Stromquist explained that they'd had to put an oxygen mask on her face and pump air into her lungs.

I was numb. I'd thought—or tried to allow myself to think—that we were past all this. Dr. Germain had violated the code when he'd pronounced her almost boring. Superstitions existed here for a reason. She'd been so close.

"On a scale of one to ten," I asked Dr. Stromquist, "how much should I be freaking?"

"Four or five," she said.

It was a serious setback. It meant that we'd reintroduced the fats too quickly, and the hole in her lymphatic system had reopened. This was going to keep her in the hospital for weeks longer. Maybe months.

"It's going to take a long time," Dr. Stromquist said.

Some babies went home on special formula, she said. Some even died. She didn't seem to be implying that was what she expected for Juniper, but it was unsettling to hear.

Every day in the NICU was a dangerous day. Every nurse knew a story of a baby who was a day or two from going home when they caught an infection and died. Dr. Stromquist was telling us that we still had many dangerous days ahead.

"Let me ask it like this," I ventured. "Which of the following holidays might she make it home for: Halloween? Thanksgiving? Christmas?"

The doctor smiled and shrugged.

When Juniper was five months old, the prongs came out of her nose. We saw her face—her whole, bare face—with its big eyes, soft cheeks, red mouth, and startled look, like, *Why are you people crying?*

Now that the fluid had been drained off her lungs, Juniper was doing all the work of breathing on her own. She still might forget sometimes, but she'd earned the right to try. The nurse told her that breathing was like riding a bike without training wheels. Tom told her the key was to keep her eyes on the road ahead and feel the wind in her hair. She kept going, going, going.

Soon, the Broviac catheter came out of her leg. Fewer and fewer tethers connected her to the hardware of the NICU. The artificial umbilicus was fraying line by line.

In early September, Nurse Carol helped me get Juniper ready for a bath. Tracy and I had sponge-bathed her before, but this would be her first warm-water immersion. Carol whipped off Juniper's diaper, peeled all the leads off her chest, disconnected the wires, and handed me a naked baby.

"What are you doing?" I asked Carol. "She's off the monitors."

She had not been this free since the moment the Labor and Delivery nurse had handed her to Gwen in the operating room. Ever since Gwen had started the first IV, Juniper had been tied to a machine. Now, I could have tucked her in one arm like a football and run for the elevators. What if I dropped her? What if she stopped breathing?

Nurse Carol had been doing this a long time.

"Are you watching your baby?" she said. "Just watch your baby."

She knew that hardware was no substitute for a mom's intuition. She knew I needed to figure out how to harness that intuition and to trust it. She knew I needed to learn to parent with no one watching. She walked out.

I wish I could remember what I said to Juniper then. I wish I could remember that candles had appeared, and soft music played, and the lights dimmed, and I rocked her and bathed her and she stared dreamily into my eyes, and I was the mom I'd always imagined I could be.

I think what really happened is that Juniper was incredibly slippery, and she kept sliding down into the shallow water, and I tried to sort of wipe her down with some gauze pads, and I wished someone would give me some grippy gloves, because what if she came this far only to be drowned by her mother in a plastic bathtub, and I must have sung her the John Prine song, the one I always sang to help her understand that the curves that flew at her in the NICU—the hard corners, the precipitous free falls, the long, grinding climbs—were pretty much the same as the ones that awaited her in life.

*It's a half an inch of water and you think you're gonna
    drown
That's the way that the world goes 'round*

None of this had unfolded as I would have scripted it. But I couldn't say it had all been bad. If we made it out of here intact, I would have to admit that this place had performed a mysterious alchemy on me. I'd do anything to spare Juniper the experience she'd been dealt, but for myself, I wouldn't change a day. I'd reconsidered every one of my values and emerged entirely reassembled. I would probably never do anything in my life as heroic as the things Tracy did in a single day. I would never have the impact of Dr. Shakeel. I had absorbed the lesson, clichéd though it may be, that it is the tiny choices we make moment to moment that determine who we are. It is, as Tom had said all along, about paying attention.

My stepson Sam had once taught me a technique handed down from a high school drama teacher. "Explode the moment," the teacher would say. It meant that every second onstage is pregnant with motive, action, tension, and purpose, and the actor needs to inhabit those moments fully and convey all of it to the audience. I'd adapted that advice for my writing students, trying to show them how to find meaning in a gesture or a glance and commit it to the page.

In the NICU, we'd been forced to explode each moment as though it were the last we might ever have. I never wanted to go back to the sleepwalker I'd been before.

I never wanted to hear "Waitin' On a Sunny Day" and think of it as just a fluffy pop song. I never wanted to see Harry Potter, who survived the darkest forces of evil with the protection of his parents' love, as a trifling figment of fiction. I never wanted to unsee my husband falling asleep on the beveled Plexiglas of the incubator, conjuring meaning from chaos. I would never forget looking up from the triage table and seeing him speckled with my blood.

Tom had shown me who he was at his core, too. I could forgive his frigid thermostat settings, his shoe obsession, his nonsensical filing system, his strange need to recite *A Christmas Carol* from memory in mid-August. Choosing him and fighting for him were the smartest things I'd ever done.

I wanted him here with me, to share in the new-parent moments. I wanted to see him camped on the floor of the nursery with a screwdriver in his hand, staring at the instructions for assembling the crib, but who was I kidding? I was the handy one in our house. I put together the crib by myself in an hour. Tom was back at work in Indiana. He was only gone two or three nights a week, but Juniper changed so fast that he'd have to scramble to catch up.

Juniper's goal now was to drink from a bottle. After being on a ventilator so long, she wanted nothing in her mouth. Tracy warned us she would probably go home on a feeding tube — lots of preemies did. It would be worth it, she said, to just get her home. I couldn't stand the thought of one more surgery, one more hole in her body. Her belly was gouged and gnarled with scars.

A speech therapist named Julie started working with Juniper, slowly at first, with just a drop of milk on a pacifier. I'd gone back to work to edit a project. The office was less than a mile from the hospital, but Juniper was more aware of my absences, so the distance felt farther. I dashed out of work at least twice a day so I could learn how to feed her. For her to be able to go home, she had to take all her milk from a bottle, and she had to do it for me and Tom, not just for the nurses.

At first, she drank just a thimbleful. I knew better than to rush and squirt the milk into her mouth. So many newborn puppies had prepared me for this. Kim showed me how to rest my index finger along her jawline and use my middle finger to support her chin. She showed me how to twist the bottle just so to remind her to keep going.

I demonstrated this to Tom when he was home from Indiana. The long-distance commute made him a poor student. He would fall asleep, and his chin would drop to his chest, and the bottle would drop to his lap.

"Tom, wake up."

"What?" he'd snap. "I've been feeding babies since before you were born."

I hit "record" on the video camera as he fed her more or less successfully and laughed when she puked all over his shirt.

"There's a book out called *Raising the Strong-Willed Child*," Tracy said. "You might want to pick one up."

Eventually, with weeks of guidance and therapy, Juniper drank a few swallows from the bottle, then a few more. We were slowly reintroducing fats into the milk. So far, she was doing fine without the chest tubes. Juniper had been in the NICU longer than any of the other ninety-six babies. Kim sat with me one night and reminded me that this place was supposed to be temporary. It was not a place for babies to grow up.

"You won't believe how she'll take off when you get her home," Kim said.

Home. My mind flashed to the house on Woodlawn Circle, the one where Nat and Sam had grown up but where I'd never felt like I belonged. Tom said I'd feel differently when I brought

Juniper there. But somehow, the NICU, the least natural environment I'd ever encountered, felt like home now.

I was learning to be a mom to a real, actual, wiggling, crying baby, and I had Tracy, Carol, Kim, and Ana Maria to help me. At night, when I was exhausted, I could hand her to Kim, who always knew how to calm her. If she felt gassy or uncomfortable, Ana Maria could fix it in an instant. I never had to stay up all night listening to her cry. If I was worried about her temperature or her color, I just pressed a button, and reinforcements appeared. I rarely asked when we could go home anymore. With Tom back at work, it was just me and her, figuring each other out. Being home alone with a newborn would be lonely. Here I was surrounded by a community of women who had every answer.

Scrunch the diaper this way, so she can close her legs all the way.

That looks like reflux; prop her up in the bed, like this.

I could not imagine leaving this place, leaving behind the reassurances of the doctors, the nurses, the monitors. Who would take care of this baby? Who would take care of me?

"Will you come, too?" I asked Kim.

One night, after dark, I held Juniper to my chest and sang to her in the blue chair. She was bundled in her blanket, alert and happy. Feeding time wasn't for an hour or so; I just told her I loved her and described the fun we would have someday. Juniper started to gnaw on my shirt. I froze, not sure at first what was happening. It was not an accidental, casual slobber. Her meaning was clear. Everyone had said breast-feeding was out of the question, after all this time. But now my baby was growing frantic, trying to eat the buttons off my shirt.

I would have given her anything. But my boob? The room was dark, and Kim was out in the hall somewhere. Juniper wasn't really supposed to have whole breast milk, with all its ominous long-chain triglycerides. But saying no seemed cruel, and how much was she really going to get, anyway? I looked around as if we were about to break a law and then unbuttoned my shirt. She latched on. I heard her swallow.

It was exactly as weird as I'd imagined it would be.

"Kim!" I wailed. "What the hell?"

Kim stuck her head inside the room. She smiled so big, she looked like she might cry.

Tom

Deep into that long summer, the rooms around Junebug filled with new arrivals. A baby girl was wheeled into the room directly across the hall. Her nameplate identified her as Eleanor, and it turned out she'd been flown in from the Caymans. Her mother was still in the hospital in the islands, but I could see the father slumped into a chair next to his daughter's incubator, his face in his hands. His hair was tousled and gray.

"What's that old-timer doing up here?" I wondered. A second later I caught my silver-haired reflection in the window and laughed.

A little boy named Freddy, farther down the hall, had also been flown in from the Caymans. His mother had delivered twins, but only Freddy had survived, and now the doctors had him on oxygen. I was sitting with Junebug early one morning, reading another chapter in book 4, when Tracy asked if I would be up for a chat with Freddy's mom.

"I think she could use somebody to talk to," Tracy said. "Somebody who's been through it."

A few minutes later, Freddy's mom showed up at the door. Amanda, cooing at Junebug, took a seat beside me. I told her our story, and she told me hers. She had gone into early labor with her twin boys on the day of their baby shower. Something had gone wrong with the supply of blood and other fluids, and one of her boys had died shortly after birth. Freddy was hanging in there, but his left leg had been so damaged that the doctors had been forced to amputate it above the knee. Amanda explained all of these things without a hint of self-pity. She had already lost one child, and now the other was fighting for his life, minus a leg. But she and her husband were grateful for Freddy and grateful to be here in All Children's. She was sure her son's chances had improved the moment he arrived on Six South.

When she left, I did not move from my chair. I'd had the impression that Amanda needed someone to cheer her up. But she had spent more time encouraging me. She had gone on and on about how beautiful Junebug was, how strong and fierce. She knew we had been in the NICU for a very long time, but when she smiled at my daughter, I saw something in her eyes that told me she was sure that Kelley and I would be taking Junebug home someday soon, just as she and her husband would take Freddy home.

Tracy returned a few minutes later but paused at the door when she saw that my cheeks were wet. "Uh-oh," she said. "I guess that wasn't a good idea, inviting her down here."

I looked at our nurse, who had saved Junebug's life more times than I could count. I was grateful she was working with Freddy.

"No, it was good," I said. "It was very good."

I had once thought of the NICU as a place suspended between life and death. But the longer we stayed, the more I realized it was also a place where I had been given another chance. Our time in Six South had forced me to hold still. It had shown me who I was, and who I was not. Junebug had given me a reason every day to wake at dawn. I wasn't nothing. I wasn't a facsimile. I was a father, and a husband, and a writer who knew beyond a doubt that stories kept us alive.

We were flying now, my little girl and I. She was sitting in my lap every morning, usually wearing a knit hat my sister Susi had made for her, adorned with a Golden Snitch, and as I read, she looked up at me and looked down at the book and reached for the pages. Though I could not prove she was smiling, her sat number told me it was true. We were sailing through book 4, spinning through the Yule Ball and watching Hermione come down the stairs for her grand entrance and shaking our heads at Ron for being such an idiot.

"Boys can be very stupid," I told my daughter.

Junebug's mind was open, which emboldened me to impart a little early dating advice. I told my daughter she didn't need to find a bad boy to tame; what she needed was a good boy with a bit of an edge. Somebody with a brain, somebody who woke up in the morning with a plan. Avoid any guy swinging nunchucks in front of a Bruce Lee poster, I told her.

One day I sat her up and looked her in the eye. She was drooling but seemed at least halfway awake.

"Listen," I told her. "I know that Disney is very, very powerful and that I won't always be able to protect you from their influence. Sooner or later, their global marketing will find you, and they will make you want to dress in pink and play princess. Your mother and I will tolerate this nonsense for a little while. You can invite me to a tea party, and I will sip from your little cup and saucer. You can even ask me to wear a tiara, and I will do it. But eventually, we will expect you to grow out of the princess bullshit."

The clot was gone, the swelling was gone, and Junebug's

bowels were healed. The apneas and the bradys still knocked her down, but these episodes were growing more rare, and she was recovering from them more quickly. The octreotide was attacking the chylothorax again. As the fluid around Junebug's lungs receded, Tracy decorated the back of the incubator with pieces of tape, each dangling like a tiny flag.

"To ward off evil spirits," she said.

One day I was singing "Hey Jude" when the speech therapist came in. Julie sat beside us, and before I knew it, she was singing along. When we got to the rounds of chanting at the end, our voices were completely in sync, and Junebug looked back and forth at us, amazed. Or maybe she was waiting for us to shut up. Her expressions were so mercurial. One second she would be beaming, and then a storm would sweep across her face.

Sometimes storms would roll through me as well, at moments I could not foresee. I was reading from chapter 23 of *The Order of the Phoenix* when I came to a scene I had forgotten. Harry, Hermione, Ginny, and Ron were visiting Ron's father in St. Mungo's, the hospital for wizards, when they ran into their friend Neville Longbottom and his grandmother. Neville was visiting his parents, who had been tortured by Voldemort's followers to the point of insanity, two shattered souls who would never recover their senses. While Harry and his friends watch, Neville's mother walks toward them wearing a nightdress, her face thin and haggard, her hair gone white. Though she doesn't speak, she motions Neville over and hands him an empty candy wrapper, one of many she has given him over the years. Neville thanks her, and she returns to her bed, humming to herself. When she's gone, Neville's grandmother tells him to throw away the wrapper. But Harry sees Neville slip it into his pocket.

The last detail crushed me. Junebug was still in my lap, but I couldn't help crying over the power flowing inside the scene—the mother longing for her child, the child longing for his mother. For the next couple of hours, I sat quietly with my daughter, grateful that she was inside this hospital, grateful that she had her mother and her father, grateful that we had her, and grateful that Kelley and I had each other.

Things were better. Kelley was looking in my eyes and talking to me again. We were laughing, and hanging out together at night, and learning how to talk about something other than the baby. Almost every day now, between the hospital and our jobs, we snuck a kiss. Eventually she confessed to me why the baby had come early—that it was likely Muppet thumping against her stomach, not the fall on the bike. I didn't care. It didn't matter.

One morning the Milk Depot called to say that they had no more room for all of Kelley's milk and that she needed to take it home. They had packed the frozen bottles—fourteen hundred of them—into giant Ziploc bags, tied them together, and loaded them onto a cart. The bags were stacked as tall as my shoulders, and both of us had struggled to push the cart onto the elevator and transfer the bounty into our 4Runner. The reality of what we were doing—pushing 300 pounds of mother's milk for a 6-pound baby—was so absurd that we couldn't help cracking up. We had bought a spare freezer just for the milk, and when we found that the freezer wasn't big enough we started laughing again. A surreal humor was seeping into our lives, a sign that we were letting down our guard. Both of us had begun to believe that our daughter was coming home. Nurses were approaching me in the hall. They were telling me that they had never seen another baby come back from the edge the way Junebug had done. Now when they heard her yelling and complaining and demanding that I pick her up, they smiled.

"Your daughter has an incredible will," one nurse said, "and that's why she's still alive." She looked toward the incubator, where Junebug was crying again. "But when she's a teenager? I'm so sorry."

Kelley

In September, orders came down to transfer Juniper to the less critical side of the NICU, the side for the feeders and growers. Some nurses called it slurpin' and burpin'.

Tracy almost never worked on the north side. Slurpin' and burpin' was not her thing. She liked the itty-bitty babies, the ones who couldn't cry or complain, the ones who needed the steadiest hands and the most exacting care. I understood. Those babies needed her. They would be lucky to have her back. But I'd mourned for weeks, fearing this day would come. I could not do this without Tracy. I couldn't leave her behind.

"It's okay," Tracy said. "I'm going with you."

No wonder she'd been hesitant to take a primary patient. For Juniper, she had come in on her days off, she had rearranged her schedule, and now she was taking her zebra clogs and her Brighton bag to the other side of the unit. She would have to care for more babies over there. The babies would talk back. They would spit up. They would leak poop out their giant Pampers. I wanted to hug Tracy, but she wasn't really the hugging type, so I just bounced a little on my toes.

If we had to go, we decided, we'd go in style. We dressed Juniper in a faux-leather jacket from Build-A-Bear and put on her Aretha Franklin inauguration hat and a new pink tutu, handmade by Tracy. We loaded a cart with her stuffed animals and blankets and books and wheeled her crib to her new room. Tracy let me carry Juniper all the way there, and as we passed the other rooms, nurses and other parents all stopped what they were doing to look. All afternoon, people filed into the new kid's room to check out the outfit. The north side was filled with unfamiliar faces. No one knew Juniper's history—not the long nights she'd lingered close to death, not the days she'd swelled beyond recognition, not the weeks she'd leaked fluid like a broken faucet. I taped the photos in sequence on a cabinet door, so they would understand.

The room across the hall from ours was a revolving door of society's ills. The babies never stayed long. One mom paraded through the NICU in oversize, extra-dark sunglasses, which she never took off. She wore stripper heels and a dress so strangely cut that I could see every inch of her swelling, tattooed breasts from the side. She spent all day gossiping on her cell phone while her baby lay in her crib, ignored.

One dad just slept in the chair, his trucker cap pulled down over his eyes, never paying the slightest attention to the newborn in the crib. Why was he here at all? I wondered. "Are you ready to take her home?" the nurse asked. "Yep," he said, but he never looked up.

One couple struggled to learn to put on a diaper. Tracy patiently walked them through the steps.

"And you know with little girls you wipe front to back, like this, okay?" Tracy said.

The baby was wailing. The mom fumbled with the diaper and scolded her daughter.

"Oh, you've got it soooo hard," she said, loud enough to be heard down the hall. "Life sucks, doesn't it? Yeah, it sucks to be you. It sucks to be you."

In these moments Tracy put on her surgical mask so the parents wouldn't catch any disapproval on her face. She assured me that the hospital social workers were aware of everything that happened on the floor. She closed the door to the room across the hall, so I couldn't stare.

"Leave it open," I begged. "Please?"

Tracy rolled her eyes over the mask.

I'd recovered, mostly, from my fear of a damaged child. Now I had a different perspective. Babies are born in all conditions, and all of them need someone to take them home and love them.

"Does that one need a family?" I always asked. "I could take another one."

Tracy knew what lurked in their genes and their cells. I couldn't imagine the dysfunction and disease she grappled with every day. She never disclosed anything about the babies' families or their health or their histories. She was a vault. But we developed a running joke every time I saw her holding another baby.

"Can I have that one?" I would ask.

"No," she would say.

I loved to be in the NICU at night, now that I worked during the day and Juniper was so alert and aware. Kim began unhooking Juniper's monitor long enough for me to put her in a baby sling and walk the halls. Breaking out of that twelve-by-thirteen room felt like breaking out of Azkaban. Juniper peeked out of the wrap in astonishment at the world, which had just opened beyond her imagining. We'd say hi to all the babies as we passed their rooms. Jersey, Dontrell, I'mya, Freddy. There were always Miracles and Nevaehs—*heaven* spelled backward.

I ached along with the babies going through drug withdrawal, their screams ricocheting through the halls. Through the blinds on their windows, I could see their heart rates soaring.

Juniper was outgrowing the hospital. She needed to sit in the sand on the beach and taste the salt in the air. She needed to grab fistfuls of grass and dog fur and dirt. She needed to feel the sun on her face and watch the rain bead on the back of her hand.

She liked it when I walked fast. Eventually I was allowed to carry her as far as the big window by the sixth-floor elevator. I held her up to it and let her look out at the lights and the moon and, in the distance, Tampa Bay.

"There's a big world out there," I told her. "I'm going to take you there."

I saw our reflection in the glass.

Juniper was taking half-ounce bottles, then full ounces, then two ounces. Slowly, she stopped having apneas. The eye doctor said that inexplicably her retinas had reversed course and were now developing as they should. She'd come as close to surgery as a baby could, and he'd never seen one improve so dramatically.

"It's a miracle," he said. "Thank your nurses."

I sat with her on the swivel chair in the corner of her room and held her tight to my chest. Then I spun her as fast as I could, clockwise and counterclockwise, because I'd read a study saying it was good for her vestibular system. Beneficial or not, she seemed to like it. I propped her in front of a mirror and worked on her tummy time, to strengthen her neck. I rotated her black-and-white flash cards of animal shapes so she wouldn't get tired of the view.

"Doing your schoolwork, Junebug?" Tracy would say.

I marveled as she learned to do the things babies do. She reached for the dancing safari animals on her mobile. She screamed when I put her back in her bed at night.

Discharge day was looming now. She was back to regular milk. All she had to do was act like a normal baby for forty-eight hours, and she could go home. Tom and I took the mandatory CPR class, practicing on inflatable babies and tossing them at each other across the conference table. I spent hours in Babies Я Us, considering waterproof crib sheets and diaper cream. In a fit of anxiety, I ordered a home monitor that would alarm if she stopped breathing in her sleep. I stocked the shelf above the changing pad with neatly folded Pampers, size P. I hung a video monitor from the ceiling above her bassinet, then rolled the bassinet into our room and parked it next to my side of the bed, where I could reach out and touch the mattress in my sleep.

I didn't tell my parents that the day was approaching. I told very few friends. I didn't want to jinx it, and I didn't want visitors. I wanted to bring her home to a quiet house, just me and Tom and the dog. I wanted to lie with her on the big bed, window light cascading across her face, and memorize her puzzlement as she beheld the ceiling fan, and maybe play a little Springsteen.

As Tom and I were checking in at the desk one afternoon, a neonatologist approached us. I flinched, braced for bad news, but he was smiling.

"I've worked here a long time, okay," Dr. Tony Napolitano said, "and there's such a thing as a miracle. And your baby is one."

Miracle. We heard that word so often now. We'd even heard it in the early awful days, when her survival was a murky improbability. Back then I'd cringed. It was an overused, Hallmark cliché of a word. It was a word people used when the truth was so much more complicated. Now, though, I didn't mind. The people who said it spoke from experience and insight I didn't have. Coming from Dr. Napolitano, it felt earned.

On matters of faith, Tom and I had little clarity. But we were forced to ask ourselves if we had been part of a miracle. If, beyond all expectation, a God that neither of us had served well had given us a gift we did not deserve.

By then, I knew some things I wished I'd known when Juniper was born. I saw cracks in the statistics that allowed room for hope. They didn't lessen the miracle, but they gave it shape and mass.

The odds Dr. Germain had quoted to us the first day had been correct: she'd had an 80 percent chance of death or significant disability. But there was another way of slicing the numbers that I had not considered until later. I should have told Dr. Germain to take death out of the statistics, because if we didn't resuscitate her, she would certainly die. So the number I needed to know was this: if we tried and she lived—as big an if as that might be—what were the odds that she could be okay? The answer was about half. That's a bet I would have taken. It would have made that long night more bearable.

All those times I had searched the statistics for loopholes, hoping to find an exemption for good parents, I would have been comforted to know that studies do show that babies with involved families have a huge advantage. I didn't learn that until Dr. Raj clued me in when she was two months old. I would have wanted to know that babies who survive three days have sharply improved odds. I would have wanted to know that studies support what we witnessed about how music and stories could reach her across the barriers of Plexiglas and narcotics. A friend shared an insight later that would have meant everything then: sound, he said, is a form of touch. I would have wanted to know the power we had, and the power she would have over us. I would have wanted to know about the gift inside each day, the terrifying ones and the merely worrisome ones, too.

None of that diminishes the miracle. Juniper astonished doctors who were not easily moved. But Tom and I were uncomfortable imagining it was as simple as God laying his lightning-bolt finger on our baby's head, passing over some other baby along the way. Passing over all those babies we saw lying under the sheets.

The things I knew with certainty were these: that back in April, a young, inexperienced nurse looked at our baby at a critical moment and saw what machines had not seen. That one of the best nurses in the hospital risked her heart and went against her own judgment when she agreed to take Juniper on. That a doctor facing an impossible decision looked into our baby's eyes and told God he was in control before ordering a risky surgery. That a surgeon thought our baby was beyond repair but somehow fixed her anyway. That a one-pound baby found the will to keep going day after day, until finally some version of the world that awaited her came into focus.

I said a prayer of thanks every day. But I believed that the miracle was all around us, in little pieces. The science that created her inside a petri dish. The obstetricians who stalled my labor. The machine that breathed for her.

Jennifer, who gave her egg. Mike, who held my hand. Tracy,

with her attention to the smallest details. Diane, with her unwavering optimism. My husband, with his faithful reading from a four-thousand-page story, and his belief that the ending was worth waiting for, and we'd all get there together.

Kim and all the other nurses who came running when I wailed, who taught me to watch the baby, not the monitor. I had wondered, once, how to mother a sci-fi baby in an artificial world. All those people taught me how. Juniper taught me how.

So if you said there was a miracle in any of that, I would say that was true enough.

I was talking about this with my friend Stephen one afternoon over Thai food. Stephen is not much older than me but is far more wise. He had been Juniper's first visitor on the day she was born, showing a willingness to engage and celebrate this baby and stand beside us in our most vulnerable moments. He had been part of the miracle, too.

He looked up over his peanut sauce and told me I had missed the point.

"Love is the miracle," he said. "The miracle is just that we are capable of loving each other. That's it."

Of course that was it. It was all a cliché, and it was all beautiful and true. Every day with Juniper had been a miracle. She'd remade our world. I was a mother now. I knew what that meant. It was not a child's imagining anymore.

Tom stood in the kitchen in his boxers, fumbling with the coffee filter.

"Honey, are you excited?" he asked.

"Yes."

It was October 25, 2011. Day of Life 196.

The house was spotless. The car had been detailed. The dog had been washed. It was our last morning alone in our house for, oh, years.

"Yes, but are you *excited?*" Tom asked. "Do you want coffee? Today she'll be crying, for us, in our house."

He paused, staring at the coffee filter. The filter for the coffeemaker with which he'd made coffee every morning for at least five years.

"I've never seen anything like this," he said.

"You've never seen a coffee filter?"

He was so tired. We'd forgotten what normal felt like. It was all going to change again anyway.

"Do I just drop it in?"

"Just drop it in."

Tracy came to the hospital in the middle of her vacation. Kim came in with tears on her face. Dr. Shakeel lifted Juniper in her arms. Ana Maria gave her one last shoulder rub. Nurses, social workers, lactation consultants, respiratory therapists, patient-care assistants, and a trainee from gastroenterology all converged on our room in Six North. Tom read from chapter 7 of book 7 of the *Harry Potter* series. Diane reminded us that she'd never doubted this day would come.

Juniper wore a red tutu and a onesie that said CHICO'S BAIL BONDS: LET FREEDOM RING. Then she pooped all over that outfit, and Tracy orchestrated an emergency bath and produced from her big bag a homemade Harry Potter onesie. That was Tracy, pulling the answer out of her magic bag one more time. Finally Kim and Tracy together disconnected the last of the wires and monitors. They peeled the leads off her chest. They unwrapped the pulse oximeter from her foot.

We buckled Juniper into her car seat and carried her out.

No wheelchair and no balloons, but that was okay. Tom and I walked side by side, Tracy beside us.

"She won't know which of us is her mom until we get to the car," I said to Tracy, not kidding.

In the elevator, we negotiated who got to carry her out. (Tom as far as the door, then me.) A couple in the elevator laughed at us. I wondered whether they were longtimers, like us. I wondered about the child they were tending to. My brain still played the game. Cystic fibrosis? Leaky heart? I remembered nights when I'd approach the building and look up at all the lighted windows and wonder about the terrible things happening inside. Worlds ending. Holes in the universe, opening.

Now I knew something I hadn't known then. Tremendous things happened here every day, too. They had been happening all this time, long before I had any reason to pay attention. This was our moment, but ours was not the only improbable child. The car seat went bump bump bump against my knee.

Juniper wore sunglasses, but I can't imagine what she must have made of it when those doors slid apart and everything opened up in front of her.

So much sun.

All that sky.

The Hatchling

Bedtime. She is warm, her head resting on her mother's arm, her right hand reaching for her father in the dark. Her breath is soft. Her eyelashes are so long they flutter against her mother's cheek.

"Tell me a story," she says. "Tell me about when I was a baby."

Always the same request. Night after night.

"When you were a baby, you were in Mommy's tummy," we tell her. "It was warm in there and safe. You liked it there. You were floating. We used to talk to you. We put our hands on Mommy's tummy, and we sang to you all the time."

"I wanted to come out."

"You did. You were kicking hard to get out. When you came out you were so little. And we were so scared, because you came out too early, and you weren't done cooking yet."

"Hey," she says, sitting up, suddenly stern. "I was not cooking."

"Growing. You were not done growing yet."

She flops back down.

We tell her about the first time we saw her, in the hospital. About Tracy and Kim and Diane and Dr. Shakeel and Dr. Germain and all the other people who took care of her. We don't tell her about how we counted her breaths, or that we still do.

"You lived in an incubator."

"Like the baby chickies."

"Just like the baby chickens."

She is four. She wakes in the night to check on her egg, which has been trying to hatch all day. We brought it upstairs so she could see it from her bed. She shines her little flashlight on the egg in the darkness.

"Hi, chickie!" she squeals. She is waving furiously.

The egg is pale green, medium-size, with a jagged hole on top smaller than a dime. One dark eye peeks out, then closes to rest. A long, yellow toe curls around the opening in the shell.

She is muddy boots, chipped fingernail polish, Eggo waffles, shrieking laughter, spilled glitter, pout-pout kisses, lost balloons. She rides horses, climbs rocks. Kicks the back of the passenger seat. Gestures wildly when she talks. Talks in her sleep, usually about Hermione.

"Watch," she says. "You might be mad, but this might be amazing."

She shames the older kids at gymnastics class with her hand-stands and hip circles. She needs a boost to reach the lowest branch of the climbing tree at preschool, but once she starts, she scurries to the top, looks down on the taller kids, and says, "You can climb like this when you're big like me."

She bottle-feeds the kittens and puppies from the animal shelter, sings to them, pulls them close for story time. She has eight chickens, which she carries around the yard and kisses good night. She puts on a black robe, waves a wand, and sorts her chickens into the houses of Hogwarts.

"You! Hufflepuff!" she shouts at Sesame, her favorite. It sounds like "Husslepuss."

She points to Crackers, the little flighty one. "You! Gryssindor!"

We took her to see Springsteen. She danced in the drop line and stood on her seat and pumped her fists in the air and sang. If the Boss saw her in the crowd, he probably wondered what kind of people would bring a four-year-old to a rock concert. But this was a promise, remember. Her sunny day.

Inside the plastic box, the baby chick strains against the hard shell. For hours, we've watched his fragile, wet body heave with exhaustion. What is it that makes him struggle so? Is it merely a buildup of carbon dioxide inside the shell, or could it be more than that? What does this baby bird, the size of a Ping-Pong ball, know of the acres of woods behind our house, brimming with bugs to chase and peck, or of the little girl who waits to hold him?

The girl pulls the blankets to her chin.

"He is going to sleep in his shell," she says. "He wants me to hold him. He already knows me. He loves me."

She yawns.

"It's just really special for me," she says.

We've asked her what she remembers, but it's hard to know. She knows the names of all her doctors and nurses. She says she remembers having a tube in her mouth, and that she did not like being born early.

Last summer, hoping to help her understand, we flew with her from Indiana, where we live now, to Florida and took her back to the NICU at All Children's. The staff set up an incubator in an empty room right across from 670, where she had spent so many weeks.

Juniper put her doll inside the incubator, reaching through the portholes to hold her little cloth hand. Familiar doctors and nurses flowed in and out of the room, delighted. Tracy and Diane showed Juniper the tiny diapers. Juniper popped a preemie pacifier in her mouth.

The lid was open on the incubator, so Juniper—always a climber—scrambled right on up inside, which made everyone laugh. She lay down and looked around. She asked Tracy to lower the lid a bit, and then to raise it back up. She stayed in the room for two hours, asking a million questions. Dr. Shakeel came by, put a stethoscope to Juniper's chest, and listened to her heart.

"You have a beautiful heart," the doctor said.

The chick shakes off the last bits of shell and collapses, damp and spent.

"Is that chicken dead?" Juniper asks.

"No, he's not dead. He's just tired."

She asks where the baby chick had been before he was in the egg. We tell her there was a time before we had a chick named Pip, and there was a time before we had a daughter named Juniper. Isn't that weird?

"He's making that noise again," she says. From inside the incubator comes a chirping. A voice of startling strength and determination. A voice declaring itself.

"It's very special for me," Juniper says again.

The Hatchling

After a while, the little chick begins to fluff up, and then to stand. We take him out of the incubator and place him in our daughter's waiting hands.

April 5, 2016
Bloomington, Indiana

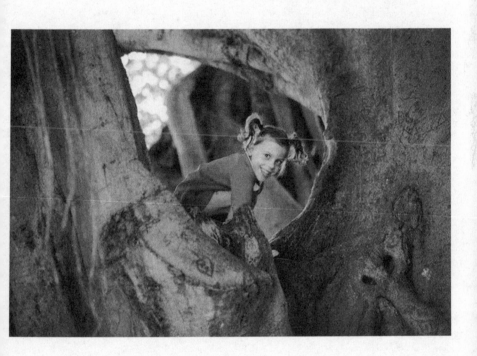

Acknowledgments

Juniper was unlucky in her timing but deeply fortunate to have been born a few floors beneath the NICU at All Children's Hospital, where she was cared for and protected and loved by more than two hundred people whose attentions made all the difference. Special thanks to Aaron Germain, Jeane McCarthy, Roberto Sosa, Gwen Newton, Whitney Hoertz, Anthony Napolitano, Debbie Lovelady, Rajan Wadhawan, Carine Stromquist, Nancy and Michael Gallant, Brooke Lowery, Donna Madden, Beth Walford, Courtney Milton, and Carol Tiffany. And to Ann Miller, who made this book possible. To Diane Loisel, who changed everything. To Ana Maria, who placed her in our arms. To Kim Jay, who stood guard in the night. To Fauzia Shakeel, who brought us all back from our darkest hour. We owe everything—every new day—to Tracy Hullett.

We could not have made it through Juniper's six months in the NICU without the countless kindnesses of our family, friends, and colleagues at the *Tampa Bay Times,* the Poynter Institute for Media Studies, and Indiana University's journalism program. Our undying thanks to Roy Peter Clark, Mike Wilson, Cherie Diez, Ben Montgomery, Lane DeGregory, Michael Kruse, Leonora LaPeter Anton, Bill Duryea, Jeff Saffan,

Acknowledgments

Stephanie Hayes, Patty Cox, Patty Yablonski, Kate Brassfield, Bruce and Suzette Moyer, Jacqui Banaszynski, Brad Hamm, Michael Evans, Stephen Buckley, Jim Kelly, Lesa Hatley Major, Tim and Bridget Nickens, Darla Raines, Neil Brown, and Paul Tash.

Thanks to Erica Allums and her crew at Banyan. A lifelong supply of sweet points to Susi French for listening and understanding through a string of terrible days. And to all the moms: Melva Benham, Sherry Wagner, Linda Rogowski, and Althea Neath. Extra thanks to Linda for going above and beyond to fact-check the waiting room decor.

A shout-out from Juniper to Dawn, Michiru, Angela and Dawson, Muppet, and Sesame the chicken.

This book sprang from "Never Let Go," a series that Kelley wrote for the *Tampa Bay Times*, with the expertise and love of many of the people named above, especially Mike Wilson, Cherie Diez, and Neil Brown. The insights of Dr. John Lantos shaped not only the story we wrote, but the story we lived. Jad Abumrad, Pat Walters, and the team at *Radiolab* helped us see that story in a whole new way, and understand that sound is a form of touch. Coaxing Kelley's series into a two-author book would not have been possible without the wisdom and enthusiasm of Roy Peter Clark and our agent, Jane Dystel, both of whom held our hands long before we realized we had a book.

We are indebted to Sara Miller for her eagle eye; to Taylor Telford for the Summer of Wonder; to the Auburn Chatauqua, especially Wright Thompson and Chris Jones, for the kick in the pants; to our colleagues and friends at Goucher College's MFA in Creative Nonfiction program, especially Patsy Sims, Dick Todd, and Susan Todd, for their unwavering kindness and encouragement; to Neil Brown and Gelareh Asayesh for telling

Acknowledgments

us to begin at the beginning; and to Tracy Behar and Reagan Arthur at Little, Brown for all their patience, guidance, and support. Special thanks, Tracy, for allowing Juniper to tear up your office.

We would not have Juniper without the kindness and generosity of Jennifer Montgomery, who is woven into every cell of our daughter and our lives. We would not have known how to keep going without Nat and Sam and their ferocious little sister.

To Juniper, we ask your forgiveness if the spotlight ever burns, and for all the days you cried because we had to work on the book. When you get big, we hope you'll read this and know how hard you fought, and how much you were loved, and we hope you will be happy at us.

About the Authors

Kelley Benham French is a professor of practice in journalism at Indiana University. A former reporter and editor for the *Tampa Bay Times*, she was a finalist for the 2013 Pulitzer Prize for "Never Let Go," a series about Juniper's survival.

Thomas French is a Pulitzer Prize–winning journalist and the Riley Endowed Chair in Journalism at Indiana University. He is the author of *Unanswered Cries, South of Heaven,* and the *New York Times* bestseller *Zoo Story.*